Handbook of
Diseases of the Breast

To our families, friends and patients.

Handbook of Diseases of the Breast

J M Dixon MD FRCS
*Honorary Senior Lecturer, University of Edinburgh
and Consultant Surgeon, Edinburgh Breast Unit,
Western General Hospital, Edinburgh, UK*

J R C Sainsbury MD FRCS
Consultant Surgeon, The Royal Infirmary, Huddersfield, UK

With contributions by

George Masterton MD FRCPsych
Consultant Psychiatrist, Royal Infirmary, Edinburgh, UK

Rhiannon Pugh MBchB MRCPsych
Consultant Psychotherapist, Fernbank Street Clinic, Glasgow, UK

Foreword by

Sir Patrick Forrest
*Professor Emeritus and Honorary Fellow,
(Department of Surgery), University of Edinburgh, Edinburgh, UK*

SECOND EDITION

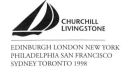

EDINBURGH LONDON NEW YORK
PHILADELPHIA SAN FRANCISCO
SYDNEY TORONTO 1998

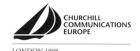

LONDON 1998

CHURCHILL COMMUNICATIONS EUROPE LIMITED

Distributed by Churchill Livingstone. A Division of Harcourt
Brace and Company Ltd, 24–28 Oval Road, London NW1 7DX

© Churchill Communications Europe Ltd

First published 1993
Second edition 1998

ISBN 0-443-06185-8

British Library Cataloguing in Publication Data
A catalogue record for this book is available from the British Library

Library of Congress Cataloging in Publication Data
is available

Note
Medical knowledge is constantly changing. As new information
becomes available, changes in treatment, procedures, equipment
and the use of drugs become necessary. The editors, contributors
and the publishers have, as far as it is possible, taken care to ensure
that the information given in this text is accurate and up to date.
However, readers are strongly advised to confirm that the information,
especially with regard to drug usage, complies with the latest legislation
and standards of practice.

Typeset by Saxon Graphics Ltd, Derby, UK
Printed in Great Britain at Biddles Ltd, Guildford

Contents

Colour plates

Foreword

The explosion of literature on the nature of breast disease, particularly breast cancer, with over 150 new published reports each month, makes it impossible for any one doctor to keep up-to-date with the literature. A difficulty which is not helped by the modern trend for large multi-author texts containing exhaustive reviews, only too often providing a source for reference, rather than coherent guidance as to the best approach. Small wonder then that doctors, other health professionals, students and patients are confused.

Michael Dixon and Richard Sainsbury have supplied a real need in writing a straightforward account of the practical issues affecting breast disorders. They have done so on a 'fast track', so that the guidelines in this small volume can be readily revised and kept up-to-date. As both authors are committed to the day-to-day management of patients in comprehensive breast units, their views and advice carry considerable authority.

The enthusiasm with which they and their publishers have tackled this project deserves congratulations and merits success.

1997   P.F.

Preface

As surgeons interested in breast disease, a stimulus to write the first edition of this book was the frustration caused by the lack of an up-to-date text dealing with the breast and the conditions which affect it. Since the first edition, there have continued to be developments in our understanding, nomenclature and treatment, and many of these have not yet reached major textbooks. The second edition of this book continues the aim of our first edition which was to produce a short didactic handbook of the breast and its diseases, setting out our current knowledge of the various conditions and how they should be managed. The aim was to produce a book which would be suitable for medical students, doctors in training — physicians and surgeons, nurses working in breast units and general practitioners. The way the first edition was received and the reviews that have been published suggest that we have, at least in part, been successful in some of our aims.

The second edition has been extensively revised and updated — large parts of the book have been completely rewritten. All this has been completed in a 3-month period and thereafter the book was revised and changes added when we received the proofs to ensure that this book reflects our current views and the up-to-date management of breast disease.

Rewriting the book in such a short period has placed considerable demands on our families and a number of other individuals. In particular, this book has only been possible because of the superb secretarial support from Monica McGill in the Edinburgh Breast Unit. JMD also acknowledges the help and support of Carol Lindsay, a Radiographer in the Edinburgh Breast Unit, who has been very helpful in identifying appropriate illustrations for the book. The help and support of Churchill Communications Europe Ltd, in particular Tara Mistry, is also acknowledged.

Psychological problems in patients with benign and malignant breast disease continue to be of great importance and we are grateful to Dr George Masterton and Dr Rhiannan Pugh who contributed Chapter 10.

We thank Professor Sir Patrick Forrest for agreeing to write the Foreword.

Finally, we would like to thank our families and friends for their continued tolerance and support throughout this and other projects.

1997   J.M.D.
                                                                 J.R.C.S.

Introduction

1. The normal breast and congenital abnormalities

THE NORMAL BREAST

Between the fifth and sixth week of human foetal development an ectodermal ridge, called 'the milk line', develops bilaterally and extends from the axilla to the groin (Fig. 1.1). Segments then coalesce into nests opposite the fifth intercostal space and in humans all but one of these nests usually disappear.

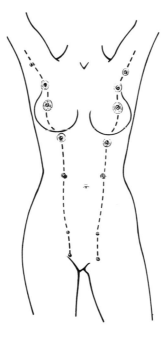

Fig. 1.1 The milk line or ridge.

BREAST DEVELOPMENT

During puberty in girls, breasts increase in size, and within each breast ducts lengthen and the branching ductules at their ends develop buds which precede the development of breast lobules. At the same time connective tissue within the breast increases in volume.

THE ADULT BREAST

The breast lies between the second and sixth ribs on the vertical axis and between the sternal edge and the mid axillary line on the horizontal axis. Breast tissue also projects into the lower axilla as the axillary tail. The functional unit of the breast is the terminal duct lobular unit (Fig. 1.2) which drains into a series of branching ducts to form between 12 and 15 major ducts which open onto the nipple. The breast does not appear to be divided into clearly defined segments, as is often described, and the branching structure of the breast is not arranged in a true radial pattern, for instance all the breast tissue at 12 o'clock does not necessarily drain into the major

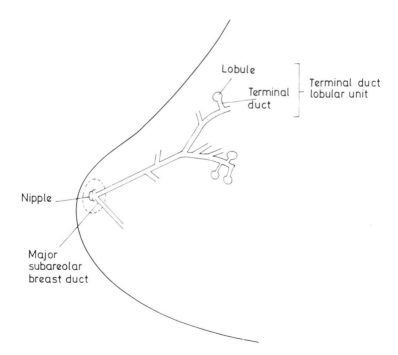

Fig. 1.2   The ductal and lobular system of the breast.

duct which opens at 12 o'clock on the nipple. The nipple and areola have certain distinctive features and the epithelium of the areola is more deeply pigmented than normal skin. At the edge of the areola there are prominent elevations formed by the openings of the ducts of Montgomery's glands which are large sebaceous glands. The subcutaneous tissues around the nipple contain smooth muscle which induces erection of the nipple.

BLOOD AND LYMPHATIC SUPPLY

The breast receives blood predominantly from perforating branches of the internal mammary artery and from branches of the lateral thoracic artery which enter through the axillary tail. The lymphatic drainage of the breast is important in relation to malignant disease. Lymph flow in the normal breast is from superficial to deep and the major drainage is then to the axilla and the internal mammary chain (Fig. 1.3). To a lesser extent, lymph also drains by intercostal routes to nodes adjacent to vertebra. The axillary nodes, which are found below the level of the axillary vein, can be divided into three groups in relation to the pectoralis minor muscle: level I

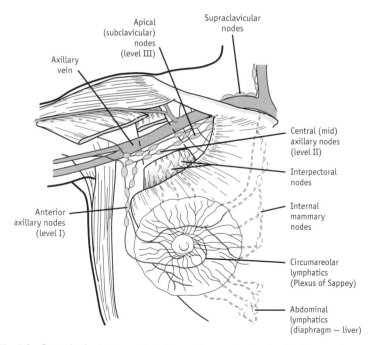

Fig. 1.3 Lymphatic drainage of the breast illustrating levels of axillary nodes.

lymph nodes lying lateral to the lateral border of the pectoralis minor muscle; level II nodes lying behind pectoralis minor muscle; and level III nodes being located medial to the medial border of the pectoralis minor muscle (Fig. 1.3). Current evidence suggests that involvement of level II or III nodes is usually associated with level I involvement. There is an alternative route by which lymph can get to level III nodes without passing through nodes at level I and that is through lymph nodes on the undersurface of the pectoralis major muscle, the interpectoral nodes (Fig. 1.3).

CONGENITAL ABNORMALITIES

One or more of the other nests persists in 1–5% of people as a supernumerary or accessory nipple or, less frequently, as a supernumerary or accessory breast. The most common sites for accessory nipples are just below the normal breast in the milk line (Fig 1.4) and the most common sites for accessory breast tissue are the lower axilla (Fig. 1.5). Accessory nipples or breasts below the umbilicus are extremely uncommon. Supernumerary nipples and/or breasts rarely

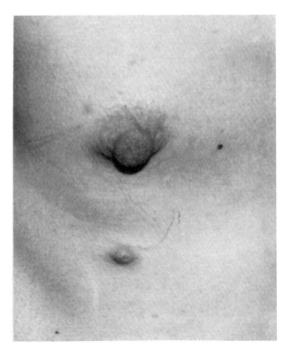

Fig. 1.4   Patient with accessory nipple.

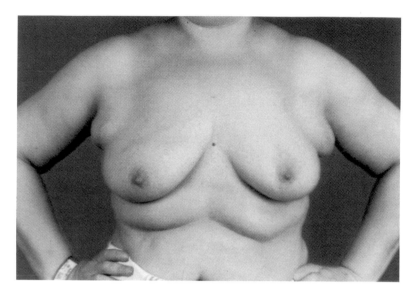

Fig. 1.5   Patient with bilateral axillary accessory breasts.

require treatment unless they are unsightly. Accessory breast tissue is subject to the same diseases found in normally placed breasts.

ABSENCE OF OR HYPOPLASIA OF THE BREAST

Introduction

One breast can be absent in isolation although it is more usual for this to be associated with pectoral muscle defects. Some degree of breast asymmetry is the norm rather than the exception, the left breast usually being larger than the right. Apart from developmental anomalies, tumours, surgery, radiation therapy and trauma can also all result in breast asymmetry. Abnormalities of the chest wall such as pectus excavatum and deformities of the thoracic spine may also result in symmetrical breasts appearing to be asymmetrical.

Treatment

True breast asymmetry can be treated by augmentation of the smaller breast, reducing or elevating the larger breast, or a combination of the two procedures.

2. Assessment and investigation of common symptoms

SYMPTOMS

An increasing number of women are consulting their general practitioner (GP) with breast symptoms. Not all such patients require referral to hospital. The important questions for the GP are:

- Is there a chance that cancer is present?
- If not, can I manage these symptoms myself?

The symptoms with which patients present to a breast clinic and their frequency are listed in Table 2.1. Painful, lumpy breasts are a common presenting symptom and a proportion of these could be appropriately managed in general practice. Only 10% of patients referred to hospital are ultimately shown to have breast cancer. Guidelines on referral of patients prepared by a Department of Health Working Party have been circulated to all GPs.

Conditions which require referral to a specialist breast clinic

Lump

- Any new discrete lump.
- New lump in pre-existing nodularity.
- Asymmetrical nodularity that persists at review after menstruation.
- Abscess or breast inflammation which does not settle after one course of antibiotics.
- Cyst persistently refilling or recurrent cyst (if the patient has recurrent multiple cysts and the GP has the necessary skills, then aspiration is acceptable).

Table 2.1   Presenting symptoms in patients attending a breast clinic expressed as a percentage (%)

Symptom	%
Breast lump	36
Painful lump or lumpiness	33
Pain alone	17.5
Nipple discharge	5
Nipple retraction	3
Strong family history of breast cancer	3
Breast distortion	1
Swelling/inflammation	1
Scaling nipple	0.5

Pain

- If associated with a lump.
- Intractable pain that interferes with a patient's lifestyle or sleep and which has failed to respond to reassurance, simple measures such as wearing a well-supporting bra and taking common drugs.
- Unilateral persistent pain in post-menopausal women.

Nipple discharge

- All women aged 50 or over.
- Women under 50 with:
      bilateral discharge sufficient to stain clothes
      bloodstained
      persistent, single duct

Nipple retraction or distortion, nipple eczema

Change in skin contour

Family history

- Request for assessment by a woman with a strong family history of breast cancer (referral to a family cancer genetics clinic where possible).

Women who can be managed, at least initially, by their GP include:

- Young women with tender, lumpy breasts and older women with asymmetrical nodularity, provided they have no localized abnormality.

- Women with minor and moderate degrees of breast pain who do not have a discrete palpable lesion.
- Women aged under 50 who have nipple discharge that is from more than one duct or is intermittent and is neither blood-stained nor troublesome.

METHODS OF ASSESSMENT

Introduction

Assessment of the breast starts with a careful history, proceeds to an examination and is supplemented by various imaging and biopsy techniques.

History

This includes details of age of menarche, age at which pregnancies occurred, age of menopause, menstrual regularity, usage of the contraceptive pill and hormone replacement therapy (HRT), family history and details of any medication. These can all be obtained by a simple questionnaire completed by the patient when waiting to be seen in the clinic. Details specific to the complaint are then sought.

The duration of the complaint is important — breast cancers grow slowly but cysts may appear overnight.

Examination

This starts with a detailed inspection in good light. The patient is examined with her arms by her side, above her head and pressing on her hips (Fig. 2.1). Skin dimpling or a change in contour should be sought. The causes of change in contour (in order of occurrence) include breast cancer, previous surgery, fat necrosis and sclerosing lesions. Deep seated lesions may only be evident in one of the three positions (Fig. 2.2). An assessment of the relative sizes (not often equal) and position of the breast can be made. Accessory nipples or breast tissue can be identified. The patient can be taught to do this in front of a mirror as part of becoming aware of her breasts and the range of normality (breast self examination is dealt with in Chapter 5). The nipple is examined for any evidence of skin changes such as eczema or Paget's disease (Fig. 2.3).

In a patient presenting with nipple discharge, it is important to determine whether the discharge is present from a single duct or whether it emanates from more than one duct. It is also important from the history to determine the volume of discharge and whether

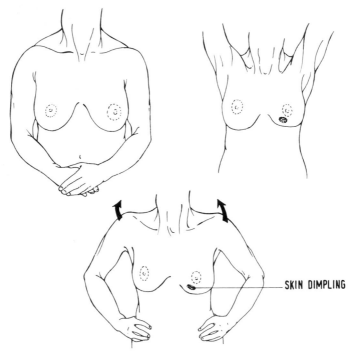

SKIN DIMPLING

Fig. 2.1   Clinical examination of the breast – positions in which breasts should be inspected.

the discharge is troublesome or persistent. During the course of examination for patients with a nipple discharge, the breast should be massaged, the nipple squeezed and a sample of the discharge assessed for the presence or absence of blood. This is achieved easily by placing a sample of discharge on a white swab. If the discharge is red or brown in colour the presence of blood should be checked by testing for haemoglobin using a dip stix technique.

Physiological nipple discharge is common; two-thirds of premenopausal women can be made to produce nipple secretion by applying suction. This physiological discharge varies in colour from white to yellow, to green to blue/black. It is often bilateral, coming from multiple ducts and is usually negative for blood on testing. Patients with multiple duct coloured or clear discharge which is not troublesome or persistent can be reassured.

The patient is then asked to lie flat and either place her arms above her head or on her hips. This spreads the breast against the

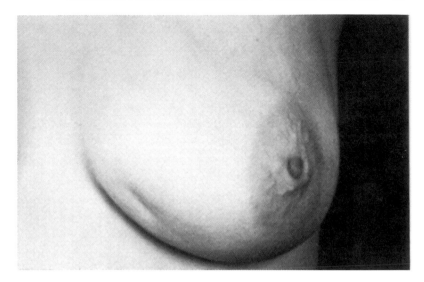

Fig. 2.2 All patients should be examined with arms by sides, above head and pressing on hips to look for changes in breast contour, as these may only be present in one of the three positions. This figure shows skin dimpling in the lower inner quadrant of the left breast with an underlying breast carcinoma.

chest wall and also allows access to the axillary tail which is otherwise covered by the patient's arm. Palpation commences with the hand held flat and aims to examine all the breast tissue rather than alighting on any dominant lesion (Fig. 2.4). Any lesion identified should then be further examined with the fingertips and assessed for deep fixation by tensing the pectoralis major by asking the patient to press on her hips. It is important when assessing the patient to determine whether any abnormality that is present is a discrete lump, that is, it stands out from the surrounding breast tissue, or whether it is a dominant localized nodular area. Young women with localized areas of nodularity should normally be assessed at a different phase of their menstrual cycle before referral to hospital by their general practitioner (Fig. 2.5). Once both breasts have been palpated the nodal areas are checked. The supraclavicular fossa and neck come first, followed by the axilla. Examination of the axillary nodes is difficult and requires the co-operation of the patient. The weight of the arm needs to be taken by the examiner to remove tension in latissimus dorsi and pectoralis major muscles, and palpation is then performed (Fig. 2.6). Nodes may easily be missed if the axilla contains a lot of fat and the correlation between clinical and pathological staging is poor.

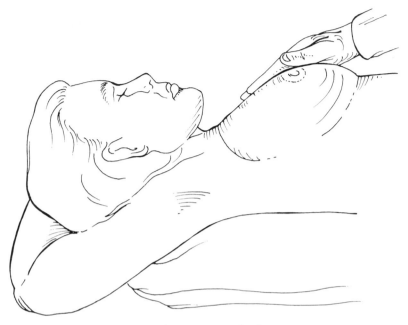

Fig. 2.4 Clinical examination of the breast — palpation.

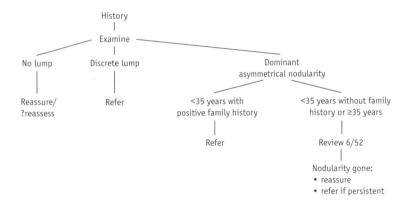

Fig. 2.5 Assessment of a breast lump by a GP.

IMAGING TECHNIQUES

Mammography

The use of X-rays to obtain pictures of the breast was described in 1930 and is now the radiological investigation of choice. It requires that the breast be compressed between two plates while the exposure

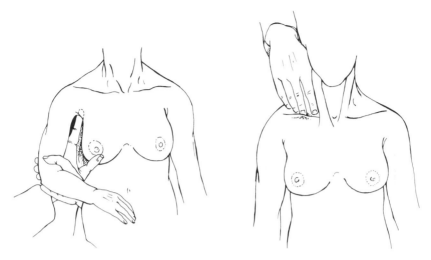

Fig. 2.6   Clinical examination of the breast — assessment of regional nodes.

is made, which may be uncomfortable (Fig. 2.7). Single views of each breast may be taken obliquely, or two views obtained (oblique and craniocaudal). With modern film screens a dose of less than 1 mGY is standard. X-ray mammography has superseded xeromammography which, although more gentle for the patient, uses significantly higher

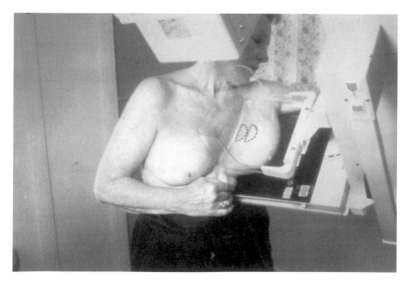

Fig. 2.7   Mammography being performed.

radiation doses. Mammography allows the detection of distortion of normal architecture, masses (Fig. 2.8) and microcalcification (Fig. 2.9). The latter may be the only indication of early disease (such as ductal carcinoma *in situ*) and is the basis for the NHS Breast Screening Programme. It must be appreciated that HRT may increase breast density (Fig. 2.10) making interpretation more difficult.

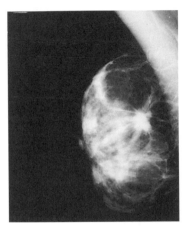

Fig. 2.8   Mammogram of a breast cancer.

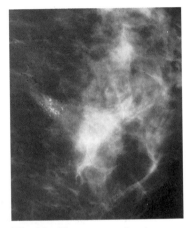

Fig. 2.9   Mammogram showing localized malignant microcalcification which was impalpable.

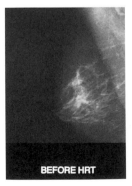

BEFORE HRT

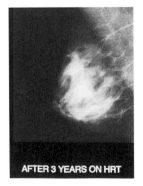

AFTER 3 YEARS ON HRT

Fig. 2.10   Effects of HRT on mammographic appearance of breast.

It is possible to carry out stereotactic cytology, core biopsy or to place a localization wire using an appropriate addition to the machine. The breast is held in a constant position and two pictures are taken at a standard angle from the vertical which allows the position of the lesion to be determined. By using needles of standard length the lesion can either be aspirated for cytological examination or marked with a hooked wire for later excision.

The breast is relatively radiodense below the age of 35 and higher exposures are needed to obtain good images. This, coupled with the relative infrequency of serious disease in this age group, means that mammography is rarely indicated in those under the age of 35. Figure 2.11 shows how the sensitivity of mammography varies with age.

Although some units allow open access mammography through GPs, it is important that those who use the service are aware of the sensitivity and specificity of mammography. The current view would be that if the patient has a condition for which mammography is indicated then hospital referral is appropriate.

Digital mammography has been developed and offers advantages in manipulating the images obtained. It allows image guided biopsies to be performed with greater accuracy.

Ductography, where contrast material is injected retrogradely into a terminal duct, has a limited, if any, role in the investigation of patients with nipple discharge.

Ultrasound

This technique uses high-frequency sound waves which are beamed through the organ of interest. The reflections are detected and turned into images. Cysts show up as transparent objects and are easily detected. Benign lesions tend to have well demarcated edges, whilst the edge is often indistinct in cancers (Fig. 2.12). There is more subjectivity in the analysis of ultrasound and hard copy is generally disappointing. Some impalpable lesions detected on X-ray mammography can be seen on ultrasound and can be aspirated or marked using this technique.

Ultrasound may be used to examine the blood flow in tumours using the Doppler technique. False colours can be generated and the technique (colour Doppler) has shown promise both in the diagnosis and management of breast masses and assessment of axillary nodes.

One disadvantage is that the equipment is expensive and not widely available.

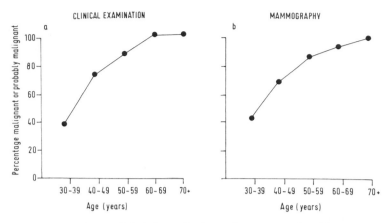

Fig. 2.11   Sensitivity of clinical examination and mammography with age.

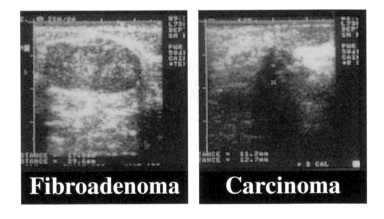

Fig. 2.12   Ultrasound appearance of a fibroadenoma and a breast cancer.

Other imaging tools

Computed tomography (CT)

This has proved disappointing for breast lesions although useful for metastatic breast cancer.

Magnetic resonance imaging (MRI)

This is a very accurate although expensive way of imaging the breast. It has a high sensitivity for the detection of breast cancer and is valuable in demonstrating the extent of both invasive and non-invasive disease in the breast. It is particularly useful in assessing the conserved breast and determining whether a mammographic lesion is due to scar or recurrence.

MRI is currently being evaluated as a screening tool for high risk women between the ages of 35 and 50.

Indications for MRI of the breast:

- Investigation of a patient who presents with axillary node metastases without an obvious cancer visible on mammogram.
- Differentiation of scar from local recurrence in patients treated by breast conservation.
- Investigation of patient with a malignant fine needle aspiration (FNA) but no mammographic or ultrasonographic lesion.
- Confirmation of extent of disease in patients mammographically suspected to have multifocal disease.
- Confirmation of suspected rupture of an implanted prosthesis.

Thermography

Breast cancers may be warmer than surrounding breast tissue and techniques for evaluating this have been tried. Thermography using heat-sensitive paper has proved disappointing but microwave (10^{-15} M) radiation has been detected and although attempts have been made to produce a brassiere with multiple detectors, currently thermography has no role in the assessment of breast cancer.

Radioisotope studies

These are mainly used to look for bony metastases. Ultrasound is more sensitive than radionucleotide scanning in assessing potential hepatic metastases. An injection of 300–600 MBq of ^{99}mTc linked to methylene diphosphonate (MDP) is given and the patient placed under a gamma camera after 2–4 h. 'Hot spots' may be identified but may require standard X-rays to confirm if the lesions seen are metastatic or degenerative. The isotope detects areas of increased osteoclastic activity and false positives are therefore common. Brain scanning can also be performed using radioisotopic techniques but CT or MRI are the imaging investigations of choice for suspected brain metastases.

Injecting technetium labelled human serum albumin into the skin overlying a breast cancer the night before surgery permits mapping of the draining nodes the next day during surgery. Using this technique it has been possible to identify with a gamma ray detection probe the draining or sentinel node. Removal of this single node provides an accurate assessment in up to 97.5% of all patients as to whether axillary nodes are involved or not. This so called sentinel node biopsy technique is gaining in popularity.

Investigations are proceeding to investigate whether measuring electropotentials over the skin of the breast provides an accurate non-invasive method of assessing the nature of any underlying breast disease. This technique is known as the Biofield Test and involves placing electrodes on the skin, rather like an electrocardiogram (ECG). Initial results are encouraging.

BIOPSY TECHNIQUES

Fine needle aspiration cytology (FNAC)

The ability to take material from a breast lesion without resorting to a formal biopsy and achieve a tissue diagnosis has been a great advance in the management of breast problems. It allows outpatient investigation with the potential to diagnose the majority of breast lesions at the patient's first visit.

FNAC requires skill in achieving adequate specimens and expertise in interpretation by the cytopathologist. In a few centres the cytologist takes the specimen, but in the majority the specimen is taken by the clinician and transported to the laboratory for analysis. To obtain reliable results care needs to be taken. A 21g (green) or 23g (blue) needle attached to a 10 or 20 ml syringe is used with or without a syringe holder. The latter may allow greater directional control whilst maintaining suction and increases the amount of material obtained, although some colleagues find it cumbersome and difficult to use. Although it has not traditionally been used in association with local anaesthetic, studies have suggested that pain and discomfort can be reduced by the infiltration of local anaesthetic into the skin and the area under the skin without reducing accuracy. The needle is introduced into the lesion (this, in itself, gives useful information as the 'feel' of a carcinoma is very different from that of a fibroadenoma) and suction applied by withdrawing the plunger of the syringe (Fig. 2.13). Multiple passes through the lesion with changes in direction allow extensive sampling. The plunger is released prior to withdrawing the needle to keep the material in the needle. The sample obtained is then expressed onto microscope slides and gently smeared. The use of heparin to pre-wet the needle has been advocated by some but seems to be unnecessary. The slides are either air-dried or sprayed with a fixative (dependant on the cytologist's preference) and later stained. Stains used include the Giemsa, Papanicolaou or haematoxylin and eosin. A report can be given in about 15 min and some units provide an immediate reporting service. This can be useful if the initial sample is inadequate as repeat specimens can be taken at the first clinic visit. The major disadvantage is that it requires the time of a dedicated technician with access to a cytologist which in many centres is difficult to justify.

Reports are either given descriptively or on a numerical score (Table 2.2). Grade 5 smears are diagnostic of malignancy. There should be few, if any, false positive results in this category and many surgeons base definitive treatment on this report. Grade 4 smears are highly suspicious for malignancy and usually 70–90% of these lesions will eventually turn out to be malignant. This category is useful as it allows the cytologist some leeway between a benign and a malignant call and is often used when only a few cells have been obtained or when the lesion is of unusual histology. Grade 3 is given if any atypical features are seen. The majority of these will still be benign although a proportion will be from carcinomas. Grade 2 reports indicate the material shows benign cells with no atypical features. Sometimes specific diagnoses can be made. A fibroadenoma, for instance, may show many naked nuclei with branched chains of cells. Grade 1 indicates that only scanty material has been obtained and Grade 0 indicates that no epithelial cells have been obtained.

In some instances it is possible for the cytologist to classify the tumour and it is also possible to perform immunohistological studies on FNAC specimens to allow assessment of oestrogen receptor levels.

The three investigations of clinical examination, imaging and sampling the lesion with a needle for cytological or histological assessment is known as triple assessment. There is strong evidence

Table 2.2 Reporting of fine needle aspiration cytology results

Grade	Result
AC0	No epithelial cells present
AC1	Scanty benign cells
AC2	Benign cells
AC3	Atypical cells present — may need a biopsy if clinically or radiologically suspicious
AC4	Highly suspicious of malignancy
AC5	Definitely malignant

that triple assessment provides more accurate diagnosis than a reduced number of tests. It certainly reduces the number of unnecessary benign biopsies. Current recommendations are that:

- All patients attending a breast clinic should have a full clinical examination. Where a localized area of abnormality is present patients should have imaging (mammography ≥35 years or ultrasonography <35 year or both) usually followed by FNAC or core biopsy (Fig. 2.14).

A lesion considered malignant on either clinical examination, imaging or cytology alone should be biopsied to provide histopathological confirmation of malignancy before any definitive surgical procedure is performed. There are no prospective data comparing diagnostic outcomes in different units. There is, however, evidence that procedures such as FNA are related to the experience of the operators. The highest sensitivities reported in the literature (and therefore the lowest miss rate and subsequently the lowest rates of biopsy) have been from specialist breast units.

Some GPs attempt aspiration of breast lumps. This allows them to diagnose those lesions which are cysts so giving the patients instant relief. As 1–3% of patients with cysts have breast cancer on clinical or mammographic examination at the time they present with their cyst, it is imperative that such patients are subsequently referred to a breast clinic for appropriate further assessment.

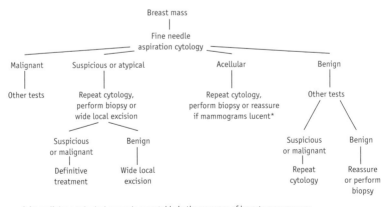

* An acellular cytological report is acceptable in the presence of lucent mammograms

Fig. 2.14   Schematic diagram for investigation of a patient who presents with a palpable breast lump. *Patients with acellular cytology and lucent mammograms can be reassured.

Unfortunately a needle introduced by a GP into a lesion which is solid can result in haematoma formation and make subsequent assessment of this lesion more difficult. In some instances a haematoma which develops after FNA can actually masquerade mammographically as a cancer. Routine aspiration of breast lumps by GPs is therefore not advised.

Nipple cytology

Scrapings from the nipple or direct impressions of the nipple onto a clean glass slide have been advocated for the diagnosis of nipple lesions. The discharge (or aspirate) from a nipple can also be examined cytologically. We have found both disappointing and currently do not use them.

Core biopsy

The aim of this procedure is to remove a small core from the mass using a cutting needle technique. A number of needles are available and these are combined with mechanical devices (Fig 2.15) to make it possible to perform the procedure with one hand, the other being available to fix the lesion being biopsied. Providing local anaesthesia is used, core biopsy actually produces less pain than FNAC. Core biopsy can be used either alone or following FNAC, if a repeat FNAC is unlikely to give sufficient diagnostic information. Local anaesthetic (1% lignocaine containing 1:200 000 adrenaline) is infiltrated into the skin, down to and around the lesion. This can make the mass more difficult to feel, but it ensures that the patient suffers as little pain as possible. Because of this, freehand core biopsy is not recommended for lesions below 2 cm. These small lesions can either be easily excised under local anaesthesia or core biopsy can be performed using image guidance. A small incision is strategically placed (11 or 15 blade) so that it can be easily removed at the time of definitive surgery, and so that the lesion can be approached at an angle of approximately 45° to the breast, to reduce the chance of damaging underlying structures in the chest or chest wall. The lesion is fixed between thumb and fingers of the left hand and the needle is introduced through the skin and breast until it abuts against the lesion. The gun is then fired and a core of tissue obtained. The core biopsy specimen is then removed from the needle and fixed in formalin, those which sink being more likely to give a diagnosis of malignancy than those which float. The needle is then inserted back into the breast and further core biopsies obtained.

Providing sufficient local anaesthesia has been given, the whole procedure should be painless and so the biopsies should be repeated until the operator is certain he has obtained a satisfactory sample from the area of concern. Frozen section reporting of core biopsies is advocated by some, but is not recommended. Bleeding is not usually a problem after core biopsy, particularly if adrenaline is added to the local anaesthetic solution, but it is appropriate to apply firm digital pressure over the lesion for several minutes. Finally the small skin incision is covered by an occlusive dressing. The result is usually available within 24–48 h. Nowadays, the procedure has a sensitivity of malignancy of over 90% but it is only of definitive value in suspicious lesions when a diagnosis of malignancy is obtained; a suspicious lesion with a benign core biopsy requires further investigation. The reporting system is different from a cytological report and is shown in Table 2.3. The essential difference is that a core biopsy should give a definite diagnosis or indicate if excision is required.

The specimen may be subjected to X-ray examination if the lesion being sampled contains microcalcifications. This ensures the correct area has been sampled.

Investigation of a patient presenting with a breast mass

All patients should be assessed by triple assessment. It is not necessary to excise all solid breast masses and a selective policy is recommended based on the results of triple assessment (Fig. 2.14). Table 2.4 shows the effectiveness of the individual components of triple assessment.

Open biopsy

If a diagnosis cannot be made by the combination of clinical examination, mammography and FNAC then an open biopsy may be necessary. Where there is a suspicion that the lesion may be malignant the excision should include a margin of normal breast tissue.

Table 2.3   Reporting of core biopsy results

Grade	Result
B1	Normal breast tissue
B2	Benign lesion
B3	Hyperplastic lesion present
B4	Severe atypia or carcinoma *in situ* requiring excision
B5	Malignant lesion

The open biopsy may be performed as either an incisional or excisional procedure.

Incisional biopsy

This procedure is rarely required as it should be possible to obtain sufficient tissue for a definitive diagnosis and immunohistochemical assessment of oestrogen receptor using a core biopsy. If an incisional biopsy is considered appropriate an incision is made directly over the lesion either along Langer's lines or along the lines of resting skin tension (Fig 2.16a and b). The incision should be made through normal skin, if necessary a small distance away from the clinical tumour mass. The incisional biopsy is usually best obtained with a knife. After securing haemostasis, the wound is closed as for excisional biopsy.

Excisional biopsy

This technique aims to remove the palpable lesion with a minimal amount, if any, of surrounding breast tissue and should be performed only if all investigations, including FNAC, suggest the lesion is benign. Lesions within 5 cm of the areolar margin can be removed through a circumareolar incision with tunnelling in the plane between the subcutaneous and breast fat, leaving an excellent cosmetic scar. For other lesions the skin incisions should either be curvilinear or follow the lines of resting skin tension (Fig 2.16a and b). Many apparently discrete lumps are nodular areas within the breast plate and these can be difficult to excise. Lesions that

Table 2.4   Accuracy (%) of the different investigations in diagnosing benign and malignant disease

	Clinical examination	US	Mammography	FNAC
% of cancers considered malignant or probably malignant (sensitivity)	88	85	88	95
% of lesions diagnosed malignant which are cancer (positive predictive value)	95	92	94	99.8
% of lesions diagnosed benign or normal which are benign (specificity)	91	88	90	95

US = ultrasound; FNAC = fine needle aspiration cytology

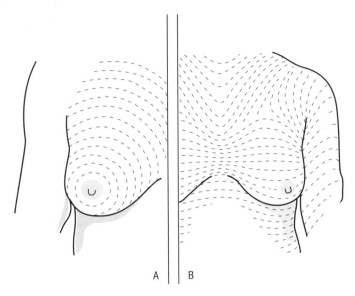

Fig. 2.16   (a) Langer's lines and (b) lines of skin tension as guides to incisions for breast biopsy.

demonstrate clinically, cytologically and mammographically to be fibroadenomas can be shelled out. Otherwise for most localized masses, the fingers of the left hand are placed on the lesion and dissection is performed with scissors, or if the tissue is dense with a knife, just beyond the tips of the fingers taking care to remove only a minimal margin of normal surrounding tissue. The size of the defect within the breast plate is an important determinant of the ultimate cosmetic result. If the lesion is grasped with tissue forceps, as is often suggested in operative texts, distortion of the lesion can make accurate excision difficult.

Tissue forceps should only be applied when the lesion has been clearly defined and has been almost completely excised. Fibroadenomas are often attached to the breast by a small pedicle which is divided prior to removal. Following excision the lesion should be fixed in formalin, unless it is considered to be suspicious at operation when it may be sent fresh. Haemostasis is secured with diathermy and drains should not normally be used. Suturing the defect in the breast frequently results in distortion and is not generally advocated. The wound should be closed in one or two layers with absorbable sutures — the lower layer being interrupted, deep, subcutaneous sutures; and the superficial layer being a continuous, subcuticular suture. The use of interrupted sutures, clips or staples produce an inferior cosmetic result and their continued use cannot be condoned.

Frozen sections

A decade ago it used to be common to see on operating lists: 'frozen section? proceed (to mastectomy)'. This is now an obsolete means of obtaining a diagnosis of malignancy and all patients should know what operation they are having when they leave the ward for the operating theatre (if not well before they are admitted for surgery). Hospitals and surgeons unable to provide a diagnosis prior to definitive treatment should not be undertaking this type of work. Frozen sections carry a higher false positive rate than FNAC and should not be used for diagnosis.

Frozen sections of the excision margins after a biopsy has been obtained are used by some surgeons to ensure completeness of the resection. Assessment of margins using this technique usually takes at least 10–15 minutes.

The use of frozen sections in the assessment of nodal status is also advocated by some. Four nodes are resected and sent for histology; if positive, a further axillary procedure is performed. While this technique is very accurate if the nodes are involved, it has a low sensitivity and up to 10% of patients classified intraoperatively as node negative will actually have evidence of nodal involvement on definitive histological assessment.

Indications for biopsy of palpable lesions

The following are definite indications for biopsy:

1. When malignant cells are obtained from a lesion that is considered clinically and mammographically benign and either a mastectomy or a wide local excision and axillary node clearance is planned. The reason is that false positive results do occur with cytology, although the positive predictive value of a malignant aspirate is over 99%. If a lesion is reported as malignant on cytology and is clinically or mammographically malignant, a patient does not require further confirmation of the diagnosis prior to definitive surgery. In lesions over 2 cm a core biopsy is most appropriate; in masses below 2 cm or those between 2 and 4 cm where a core biopsy fails to confirm malignancy, then a wide local excision should be performed. For lesions over 4 cm an incisional biopsy is indicated.

2. When a lesion is considered suspicious of malignancy on clinical examination, mammography or cytology, for lesions over 4 cm a core biopsy may provide diagnostic information, but for small lesions a wide local excision is usually performed as it is both therapeutic and diagnostic.

3. In cystic disease when a cyst contains evenly blood stained fluid, when a cyst persistently (greater than twice) and rapidly refills or where there is a persistent residual mass after aspiration (such a lesion must have been present on at least two occasions and have been investigated by FNAC) these patients should have the cyst and/or persistent mass excised. This is because cancers both intracystic and adjacent to cysts do occasionally occur. A wide excision is the surgical treatment of choice so that if the lesion is malignant the procedure is likely to be therapeutic.

4. A discrete breast lesion, even when considered to be benign on all modalities of investigation, should be removed by a simple excision biopsy if the patient requests removal. A lesion which is considered to be a fibroadenoma on all modalities of investigation can be 'shelled out'. Only a small minority, 10–20% of patients, who are informed their lesions are benign request excision.

   Some authors have suggested that all symptomatic patients over a certain age should have their lesions excised, based on the knowledge that as the age of the patient increases, so the chance it is malignant also increases (Fig. 2.17). This approach is illogical as numerous benign lesions, many of which are palpable, are being identified during breast screening and are not being routinely excised. It is, however, useful to have guidelines for junior staff in breast clinics and it is not unreasonable to advise excisional biopsy of discrete breast masses in symptomatic women over the age of 40 unless there is unequivocal evidence that the lesion is benign (e.g. mammography showing a calcified fibroadenoma or lipoma and benign cytology).

5. Patients with large primary breast cancers, those with locally advanced breast cancers, and those who present with metastatic breast cancer, require a core biopsy or rarely an incisional biopsy to establish a diagnosis.

It has been advocated that all patients undergoing surgical drainage of a breast abscess should have a biopsy of the abscess cavity. Performing aspiration in all masses which might be infective permits early identification and investigation by FNAC of those

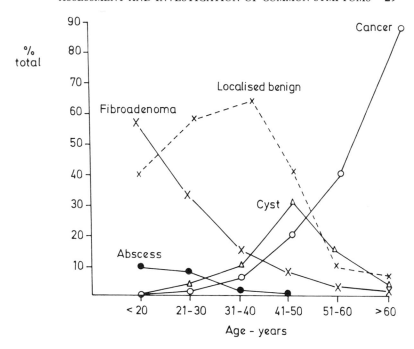

Fig. 2.17 Percentage of patients in 10-year age groups with a discrete breast lump who have common benign conditions and breast cancer.

lesions which are solid, such as inflammatory carcinomas, and obviates the need for biopsy in this condition.

Assessment of patients with mammographically detected impalpable lesions

This group has become more frequent as the Screening Programme has progressed. One important distinction between these women and those presenting to the symptomatic breast clinic is that they are not 'patients'. They are essentially well (if worried) and extra reassurance is often necessary. In every case a definitive diagnosis and plan of action need to be formulated as uncertainty is a major component of worry.

Examination needs to be carefully performed as subtle changes can be seen with even the smallest lesion. Localization of the abnormality with ultrasound or stereo X-rays may be needed, as may admission for a localization biopsy. The woman only becomes a patient when admission for diagnosis or treatment is needed. The number of women recalled for further X-rays at 6 months or a year needs minimizing.

Impalpable lesions

These are detected by mammography performed either during the investigation of symptomatic women or as part of routine breast screening. Patients with such lesions should be assessed by clinical examination, magnification mammography and ultrasound. Thereafter those which are truly impalpable and still considered suspicious of malignancy should have aspiration cytology or core biopsy performed using ultrasound or stereotactic guidance. This identifies some lesions as benign and these do not require further investigation.

Technique for excision of impalpable lesions

The lesion is localized prior to operation by the radiologist using one of a number of techniques which may include skin marking, injection of dye and contrast (the double dye injection technique), injection of carbon particles, the injection of 0.06mg of ^{99m}Tc-labelled human serum albumin or insertion of one or more hooked wires (Fig. 2.18). The most commonly used method is insertion of a hooked wire placed using either ultrasound or stereotactic guidance. There are a variety of wires available. The more modern wires are thicker in their distal portion, and proximal portion or the wires are provided with depth indicator crimps and/or a blunt cannula which can be used to stiffen the wire and make the tip palpable.

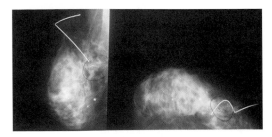

Fig. 2.18   Stereotactic-guided wide local excision of an area of microcalcifications.

Following placement of one or more wires, true lateral and cranio-caudal mammograms are taken and these films are discussed by the surgeon and radiologist prior to operation. The aim is to make a skin incision directly over the site of the lesion. This can be achieved either using the stiffening device, provided with some wires, by asking the radiologist to mark the skin directly over where the lesion is, either by visualizing the lesion itself or localizing the tip of the wire on ultrasound. If the surgeon is very experienced, it is possible to estimate from the mammograms exactly where the lesion is situated in the breast.

The incision is deepened and dissection then proceeds in such a direction so that if a single wire is being used the surgeon can identify the wire before it enters the lesion; for instance if the mammographic abnormality is being localized with the breast in the craniocaudal position, then dissection proceeds superiorly. If the lesion to be excised is widespread, as in some patients with microcalcification, the aim should be to perform an adequate excision. If one is using a dual calliper wire, it is possible to determine exactly where one is along the length of the wire by identifying the site of the change of calibre. Once the wire is identified it can be divided with sterile wire cutters and the proximal part removed. It is important not to place tension on the distal part of the wire and the wire itself should not be grasped as this may dislodge it. It is usually possible, however, to place tissue forceps on the tissue around the distal part of the wire.

Using the mammograms as a guide, a block of tissue is excised. If the operation is a definitive procedure for cancer, then the excision usually includes the full thickness of the breast down to the pectoral fascia. Some units use two or more wires placed peripherally around the mammographic lesion to assist in complete excision. Tissue is removed incorporating the wires and thus the mammographic lesion. The portion of tissue removed should be orientated, preferably with ligaclips as these are radio-opaque. One technique is to place one ligaclip on the anterior margin, two on the medial margin and three on the inferior margin, following which the specimen is X-rayed. Although it is suggested that specimen X-rays should be taken in a Faxitron, the best quality specimen X-rays are obtained using compression in a mammogram machine. Specimen X-rays must be inspected prior to wound closure to check the lesion has been excised. Orientation of the specimen has the advantage of allowing further tissue to be excised if the mammographic abnormality approaches any resection margin.

Close co-operation between the surgeon and the pathologist is required to identify the nature of the lesion and the adequacy of the excision margins. If the abnormality is not present in the first specimen, then the surgeon should re-inspect the mammograms and further tissue is then excised and X-rayed. Failure to remove the lesion after three portions of tissue have been excised, should lead to the termination of the procedure. Thereafter follow-up mammography is performed and, if appropriate, the patient should have a second localization procedure. Having excised the mammographic lesion one can mark the margins of the cavity in the breast (superior, inferior, medial and lateral) with ligaclips if a definitive wide excision of the lesion is being performed. This is of value during follow-up mammography. Haemostasis is secured with diathermy and the wound closed in layers.

Indications for excision of impalpable lesions

The decision as to which lesions should be excised depends on the radiologist's degree of suspicion and the result of stereotactic FNAC (Fig. 2.19). Lesions which may require excision include:

- A localized soft tissue mass lesion.
- An area of architectural distortion or parenchymal deformity (this includes stellate lesions).
- Clustered areas of microcalcification.
- A combination of the above features.

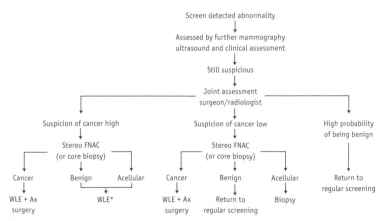

Fig. 2.19   Role of stereotactic fine needle aspiration cytology (stereo FNAC) in assessment of impalpable mammographically detected suspicious lesions. Ax = axillary, WLE = wide local excision, *extent of surgery dependent on degree of mammographic suspicion.

Recently a number of authors have questioned the value of image guided FNAC and have advocated the use of core biopsy. It is likely that the best results from impalpable lesions are obtained from a combination of core biopsy and FNAC. It is clear that the sensitivity of FNAC in impalpable lesions is less than that for palpable lesions, but it is easy to perform and can be reported quickly.

Type of anaesthetic for breast biopsy

All biopsy procedures can be performed under general or local anaesthesia; and the majority of simple excision biopsies should be performed under local anaesthesia. Although this is standard practice in the USA and in Scandinavia, many centres in the UK still advocate general anaesthesia for these operations which is difficult to defend, because local anaesthesia is acceptable to patients and more cost effective.

Intravenous sedation with midazolam makes the procedure more tolerable for anxious patients. Having palpated and identified the lesion to be removed, it should be marked on the skin either with an indelible marker or, if the skin incision is to be placed directly over the lesion, the skin can be scratched gently with the tip of a needle. This is important because once local anaesthetic has been infiltrated the lesion may be difficult to define. A 1% solution of lignocaine containing 1:200 000 adrenaline is infiltrated down to and around the lesion. During operation diathermy is utilized to secure haemostasis as for general anaesthesia.

It is current practice to perform the majority of excision biopsies under local anaesthesia, and the majority of wide local excisions and needle localization excisions under general anaesthesia. For these latter procedures it is important to be able to clearly define the margin between normal and abnormal breast, which is easier when the tissues are not swollen and distorted with local anaesthetic. Local anaesthesia is used in those patients who are unfit for general anaesthesia or where there is a specific patient preference.

Morbidity of breast biopsy

A breast biopsy performed for what is subsequently shown to be benign disease is not without morbidity. Immediate postoperative complications include haematoma formation and wound infection (in approximately 2% and 4% of patients, respectively). The incidence of these complications is not influenced by wound drainage or whether the operation is performed under local or general anaesthesia. Wound infection appears related to the nature of the underlying disease process and is most common following surgery for periductal mastitis, a condition from which both aerobic and anaerobic organisms have been isolated. A diagnosis of periductal mastitis can usually be made on the basis of the history and FNAC, and a biopsy is rarely indicated to establish the diagnosis. Operative procedures performed in patients with periductal mastitis should therefore be performed under antibiotic cover with Augmentin or a combination of cephradine and metronidazole.

Women undergoing breast biopsy suffer significant anxiety even when informed that the lesion is likely to be benign. This anxiety can be kept to a minimum by ensuring that the histological diagnosis is given to the patient as soon as it is available, which should certainly be within 10 days of the operative procedure. In the decade after breast biopsy for benign disease, 10% of patients develop a further breast mass at the biopsy site and a further 10% experience breast pain specifically related to the biopsy wound. A number of other women develop unsightly scars, either as a consequence of the postoperative complications of haematoma formation or wound infection, or because they produce hypertrophic or keloid scarring.

It has not been generally appreciated that breast biopsy is associated with such significant morbidity, as no study has followed up groups of women for long periods after these operations. Because of this potentially significant morbidity, it is essential to keep the number of biopsies for benign disease to a minimum and a currently acceptable ratio of benign to malignant lesions in symptomatic practice is 1:1. In screened women most screening centres have managed to reduce the ratio to one benign biopsy for every two cancers.

OTHER DIAGNOSTIC TECHNIQUES

Microdochectomy

This operation involves removal of a portion of a diseased duct for pathological assessment. The indications for microdochectomy are:

- Bloodstained nipple discharge from a single duct.
- Persistent or troublesome nipple discharge from a single duct.
- Periductal mastitis involving a single duct.

This operation is best performed under general anaesthesia. The infiltration of local anaesthetic distorts the subareolar ducts and makes dissection of these ducts difficult. Patients having surgery for periductal mastitis should have perioperative antibiotics, either co-amoxyclav or a combination of metronidazole and erythromycin.

Technique

After the skin has been prepared, a probe is placed through the discharging duct. Some surgeons make an incision directly across the nipple across the probe. It is more traditional to make a circumareolar incision and this probably results in a better cosmetic result. If the discharging duct is central, then the incision should be circumareolar and based at six o'clock. Otherwise a probe is passed through the discharging duct and palpated under the areola and then a circumareolar incision is made directly over the probe. The incision is deepened and the ducts underneath the nipple identified. The probe is usually palpable in the diseased duct and, having identified the abnormal duct, it is followed down into the breast tissue and approximately 2 cm portion of duct excised.

NIPPLE ABNORMALITIES

Changes in the nipple can occur with both benign and malignant disease, and include nipple inversion/retraction, nipple discharge and skin changes involving the nipple and areola.

Nipple inversion/retraction

Nipple inversion is described when the whole nipple is pulled in, and nipple retraction is described when only part of the nipple is pulled in, usually at the site of a single duct to produce a slit like appearance of the nipple. These changes can be congenital or acquired. The acquired causes in order of frequency are: duct ectasia, carcinoma, periductal mastitis and tuberculosis.

Investigations

All patients with acquired nipple inversion or retraction should have a full clinical examination and if the patient is over the age of 35 a mammogram.

Management

- If no palpable mass or mammograms are normal/benign — surgery not indicated unless for cosmetic reasons.
- If mass palpable or mammographic abnormality is evident — FNAC or biopsy and duct excision are indicated.

Nipple discharge

The causes of nipple discharge in order of frequency are: physiological, duct papilloma, duct ectasia, periductal mastitis, cancer and galactorrhoea. Nipple discharge can be from single or multiple ducts. Single duct discharge is more likely to be serious than multiple duct discharge. Physiological discharge is very common and can be obtained by massage of the breasts in up to two-thirds of patients. The amount of discharge is variable and is, characteristically, intermittent from multiple ducts and usually requires massage to produce it.

Milky discharge from a single duct is common and usually physiological. Galactorrhoea occurs from multiple ducts in both breasts and is usually associated with a raised plasma prolactin level. Bromocriptine is effective in stopping this milk flow but should be used after exclusion of a pituitary tumour (galactorrhoea and a prolactin greater than five times the upper limit of normal need investigation).

A plan for the investigation of nipple discharge is shown in Figure 2.20.

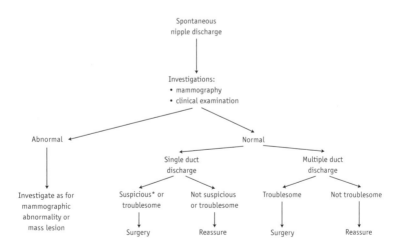

* Bloodstained or persistent

Fig. 2.20 Schematic diagram for investigation of a patient with nipple discharge. Total duct excision is recommended for patients with multiple duct nipple discharge.

TOTAL DUCT EXCISION

Indications

- Multiple duct discharge.
- Nipple inversion.
- Surgery for periductal mastitis. This can be patients who have had recurrent periareolar sepsis or can be part of an operation to excise a mammary duct fistula.
- Persistent normo-prolactinaemic galactorrhoea not responding to antiprolactin drugs such as bromocriptine or cabergoline.

Antibiotics

All patients having operations for periductal mastitis should have perioperative antibiotics (see Microdochectomy).

Technique

A circumareolar incision based at 6 o'clock is used for total duct excision. The total length of the incision should occupy less than 25% of the total circumference of the areola.

Procedure

The incision is deepened and the plane between the subcutaneous fat and the breast fat is identified and developed. A pair of dissecting scissors are then passed under the areola just peripheral to the breast ducts and a plane developed down each side of the breast ducts. The dissection is continued behind the nipple so that an artery forceps can be placed around the ducts and these brought into the wound. The ducts are then ligated if the operation is being performed for galactorrhoea or otherwise divided with scissors or a knife. If there is nipple inversion, division of the ducts should be at the lower edge of the artery forceps. This is important because it is possible to inadvertently excise a portion of nipple skin in such instances. It is always possible to trim the ducts behind the nipple at a later stage. From the central core of ducts, 1–2 cm are excised and sent for histology. It is not necessary to excise more than a 2 cm portion of duct tissue or to ligate the ends of the divided ducts in the breast tissue unless the operation is being performed for persistent galactorrhoea which is not responding to antiprolactin drugs. In this instance, the ducts themselves are ligated and divided from underneath the nipple but no actual duct tissue needs to be excised. Haemostasis is secured with diathermy. It is not usually necessary to place any sutures in the breast tissue. If it is felt necessary to buttress the tissues underneath the nipple, then a series of interrupted dissolvable sutures can be placed to approximate the breast tissue. For patients with periductal mastitis it is imperative that all diseased ducts are removed *in toto*. To achieve this the area behind the nipple should be inspected closely and any duct which contains granulation tissue must be excised. For patients having a total duct division and ligation for normo-prolactinaemic galactorrhoea not responding to appropriate drugs, the ducts are divided as described above and the distal ducts ligated with a single suture.

It is important at the end of this procedure to leave the nipple satisfactorily everted. Having identified and divided all the subareolar ducts it is usually possible to manually evert the nipple by placing the tip of the little finger underneath the nipple. If there is scarring in the nipple region which stops the nipple being everted, then any tight bands need to be divided. Only rarely is it necessary to suture evert the nipple. The problem with this latter approach is that the nipple will remain everted at all times and this looks unnatural. Drains are rarely, if ever, required after total duct excision. The wound is closed in layers with absorbable sutures.

Complications

Complications that have been reported include:

- Necrosis of the nipple. Patients at risk of this are those who have had multiple previous nipple operations. It is a rare complication in experienced hands. The nipple usually re-epithelializes with time.
- Loss of nipple sensation. This affects as many as 30% of patients undergoing this operation and all women should be warned about this complication. The amount of dissection close to the nipple should be minimized. It is only in women with recurrent infections and periductal mastitis where removal of all diseased ducts and dissection very close to the nipple are necessary. Studies have shown that patients who have pain before operation, patients with periductal mastitis and those who smoke are at most risk of loss of nipple sensation. Patients with inverted nipples who have their nipple everted do have improvement in nipple sensation so it is important during this procedure to ensure that the final position of the nipple is satisfactory.
- Recurrent discharge. This can be due to an incomplete total duct excision although occasionally it is due to the cavity

behind the nipple filling with serous fluid which then drains out through the divided nipple ducts.

- Recurrent infection. Even after total duct excision, some patients with periductal mastitis will develop recurrent infection and develop a mammary duct fistula. This is due to diseased ducts being left attached to the under surface of the nipple. A further procedure to excise residual duct tissue is usually required.

Changes in skin of nipple and areola

These can be due to eczema, Paget's disease or can occur as a direct result by infiltration of an underlying carcinoma. Patients should have the same investigations as for nipple inversion/retraction.

Management

- Where there is a mass lesion or mammographic abnormality detected this should be appropriately investigated.
- If there is no mass lesion but Paget's disease is considered a possible diagnosis then a portion of the nipple or areolar skin should be excised under local anaesthetic and submitted for histological examination.
- Eversion of the nipple can often be satisfactorily performed under local anaesthesia by incising the ducts and loosely placing two horizontal mattress sutures of chromic catgut to maintain eversion whilst healing occurs. If the nipple inversion is marked and long-standing, a total duct excision is required to evert the nipple.

Non-malignant breast disease

3. Benign breast conditions

INTRODUCTION

Benign conditions of the breast are important because:

- They are more common than breast cancer and so account for the majority of attendances to a GP and thus of hospital referrals.
- They can be difficult to differentiate from breast cancer.
- Incorrect diagnoses and inappropriate treatment of benign conditions are associated with significant morbidity.

Patients with benign breast conditions present with a lump, breast pain, nipple retraction or discharge, or are referred with a clinical or radiological abnormality found during breast screening. Most benign disorders arise on the basis of dynamic changes which occur in the breast through the three main periods of reproductive life: development (and early reproductive life), mature reproductive life and involution. The majority of benign conditions which affect the breast during these three periods can be considered as part of a spectrum from normal to overt disease. In between these extremes there are conditions which occur so frequently that they are most appropriately considered as aberrations rather than diseases (Table 3.1). The fact that there is a spectrum of change does not imply that these commonly occurring aberrations actually develop into disease.

ABERRATIONS OF NORMAL DEVELOPMENT AND INVOLUTION (ANDI)

Common conditions occurring during the stage of breast development which are best considered as aberrations of normal breast development include excessive breast enlargement during puberty (known as juvenile or virginal hypertrophy) and fibroadenoma.

Table 3.1   Aberrations of normal development and involution

Age (years)	Normal process	Aberration
<25	Breast development	
	lobular	Fibroadenoma
	stromal	Juvenile hypertrophy
25–40	Cyclical activity	Cyclical mastalgia
		Cyclical nodularity
		(diffuse or focal)
35–55	Involution	
	lobular	Macrocysts
	stromal	Sclerosing lesions
	ductal	Duct ectasia

After the stage of breast development the breast undergoes periodic changes through successive menstrual cycles. Aberrations which occur during this period include breast pain and lumpiness or nodularity. In the past, specific terms such as fibrocystic disease and fibroadenosis have been used for painful lumpy breasts but these terms are no longer considered appropriate. The reason for this is that there is a very poor correlation between the presence of localized nodularity and pain and discomfort, and what is going on at the pathological level. Breast involution starts in the fourth decade of life and includes: the development of small breast cysts (microcysts); focal areas of change in the normal epithelium lining breast ducts and lobules to sweat gland-type epithelium (apocrine change); an increase in the amount of fibrous tissue within the breast (fibrosis); an increase in the number of glandular elements within breast lobules (adenosis), and some increase in the number of cells lining the terminal duct lobular unit (minimal hyperplasia). Aberrations of this involutionary process include the formation of large breast cysts which present as palpable breast masses and excessive fibrosis which give rise to a series of abnormalities including the formation of radial scars and sclerosing lesions. Only when the epithelial proliferation within the breast lobules is excessive (moderate and florid hyperplasia) or is associated with atypical changes within the proliferating cells (atypical hyperplasia) are these changes considered as true disease.

JUVENILE HYPERTROPHY

Prepubertal breast enlargement in the absence of other sexual maturation is a common occurrence. Only if associated with other signs of sexual development is it an indication for investigation. Uncontrolled overgrowth of breast tissue occasionally occurs in adolescent girls whose breasts initially develop normally at puberty and then continue to grow often quite rapidly. This condition is called virginal or juvenile hypertrophy although it is not really hypertrophy; the histological features are an overgrowth of periductal connective tissue with proliferation of, and an increase in, branching of breast ducts without evidence of lobule formation. These appearances are no more than an exaggeration of the structure of a normally developing breast and this is why this condition is best considered an aberration of normal breast development. No endocrine abnormality can be detected in these girls.

Presentation

Patients present with a variety of symptoms: social embarrassment; pain; discomfort; inability to perform daily activities, such as regular exercise and walking down stairs; back and shoulder ache, and pain and discomfort directly under where the bra strap passes over the shoulder, where there is a characteristic indentation.

Treatment

Surgery significantly improves quality of life for many patients and should be more widely available. The aim of surgery is to reduce the size of the breast (reduction mammoplasty).

FIBROADENOMA

Although considered in most textbooks as benign neoplasms, fibroadenomas are best considered as aberrations of normal development because:

- Fibroadenomas develop from a whole lobule whereas neoplasms arise from a single cell.
- Fibroadenomatoid changes in lobules are common findings in the breasts of young women.
- Fibroadenomas show the same hormonal dependence as the remainder of the breast, for instance they lactate during pregnancy and involute during the perimenopausal period.

Incidence

Fibroadenomas account for approximately 12% of all palpable symptomatic breast masses. They are said to occur more frequently in Negro populations. The frequency with which they cause a breast lump in different ages is shown in Figure 2.17 (see page 29); they are a very common cause of a breast lump in women aged 15–25 years, but still account for 15% of all discrete lesions in women aged 30–40 years and are in fact a more frequent cause of a breast lump in this decade than cysts. Thereafter they are less common.

Classification

There are four separate entities of fibroadenoma: common fibroadenoma, giant fibroadenoma, juvenile fibroadenoma and phyllodes tumours. Fibroadenomas are characteristically classified by pathologists as intracanalicular or pericanalicular, but this histological distinction has no clinical relevance and the terminology can be abandoned. There is no universally accepted definition of a giant fibroadenoma but most consider that a fibroadenoma must measure over 5 cm in size to qualify for this definition. This type of fibroadenoma may or may not have a different behaviour to an ordinary fibroadenoma. The juvenile fibroadenoma occurs in adolescent girls and is rare. Most juvenile fibroadenomas undergo rapid growth and tend to be more cellular than ordinary fibroadenomas. These three entities are treated in an identical way.

Phyllodes tumours are distinct pathological entities and, although they cannot always be differentiated from fibroadenomas clinically, their histology and behaviour are such that they should be classified separately. Figure 3.1 shows a giant fibroadenoma prior to removal.

Presentation

Fibroadenomas usually present as a palpable breast lump, although they may be detected at screening. The majority are found in the upper, outer quadrant where most breast tissue is located. On examination they are usually well circumscribed, firm, mobile, discrete breast lumps and can occasionally be multiple or bilateral. A fibroadenoma is sometimes referred to as a 'breast mouse' because of its mobility within the breast tissue.

Diagnosis

Among the discrete breast masses thought clinically to be fibroadenomas, 5% subsequently turn out to be carcinomas and clinical diagnosis may be incorrect in up to 50%. All discrete mobile lesions should therefore be fully investigated by triple assessment — mammography (if the patient is over the age of 35 years), ultrasonography (this is useful for women under the age of 35 and also for older patients with dense mammograms) and fine needle aspiration cytology (FNAC). Mammography can, in some instances, provide a definitive diagnosis of fibroadenoma when a well-defined lesion is seen containing characteristic coarse calcification. It is now accepted that it is possible to make a definitive diagnosis of a fibroadenoma by a combination of clinical examination, ultrasound (Fig. 2.11A, see page 18) and FNAC.

Natural history

Current studies suggest that less than 5% of fibroadenomas increase in size and a third get smaller or disappear over a 2-year period. The remainder stay the same size but become clinically less distinct with time.

Management

It is routine practice in almost all units to remove those fibroadenomas over 3 or 4 cm in size. As fibroadenomas are benign and few increase in size, once a definitive diagnosis is established by a combination of clinical examination, ultrasonography and FNAC, a choice of treatments can be offered. The patient can be given the option of excision, performed under local or general anaesthetic, or observation which consists of a single follow-up ultrasound at 6 months to check the lesion has not increased in size. Some believe that observation is only appropriate in women under the age of 40 because of the possibility of missing a breast cancer in older women. The majority of women, given the option of observation or excision elect to keep their breast lumps. If access to good quality cytology and ultrasonography is not available, it is wise to excise all fibroadenomas to be certain that no malignant lesions are missed.

Phyllodes tumours exhibit a spectrum of behaviour ranging from benign to malignant, with a close correlation between the histological appearance and their subsequent behaviour. Only rarely do they metastasize and the main problem is of local recurrence. Treatment is by wide excision which, in some instances, means a mastectomy (which may be of the subcutaneous variety).

Relationship to breast carcinoma

Breast cancer is no more likely to develop in a fibroadenoma than in any other part of the breast. A group of relatively uncommon pathological lesions are known as complex fibroadenomas and appear to be associated with a slightly increased risk of breast cancer (Table 5.2).

MASTALGIA

Mastalgia, or breast pain, alone or in association with lumpiness, is the most frequent reason for a breast-related consultation both in general practice and in specialist breast clinics. It is best classified as non-breast mastalgia, cyclical and non-cyclical mastalgia.

NON-BREAST MASTALGIA

Conditions which have no association with either the breast or the chest wall sometimes present with apparent breast pain. A full history and careful clinical examination are required to demonstrate that the pain is arising from other organs. Non-breast mastalgia can be caused by angina, cholelithiasis, degenerative disorders (such as cervical spondylosis), hiatus hernia, nerve entrapment syndromes (such as in carpal tunnel or cervical rib) and oesophageal lesions — particularly achalasia, pleurisy and pneumonia or pulmonary tuberculosis.

CYCLICAL MASTALGIA

Frequency

The exact incidence of cyclical mastalgia is not known but, when directly questioned, 66% of a group of working women and 70% of a screened population admitted to having had recent breast pain, with symptoms being severe in up to one-third. Breast pain is the main presenting symptom in about 50% of patients attending breast clinics. Classically women report that they have heightened awareness, discomfort, fullness and heaviness of their breasts during the 3–7 days which precede each menstrual period. During this period women often report that their breasts increase in size and that they develop areas of tender lumpiness. Following the commencement of menstrual flow these symptoms disappear. Some patients report extreme discomfort during these few days while others report pain and discomfort which last much longer than a few days and which can start within a few days of cessation of menstruation and continue until the next period. The frequency of mastalgia suggests that it should not be considered as a disease but is best considered as an aberration of normal cyclical changes within the reproductive years. The impact of mastalgia on quality of life is often underestimated by the medical profession. Mastalgia is very uncommon as a presenting feature of breast cancer.

Aetiology

Mastalgia shows many features which suggest that it has a hormonal basis, but no consistent hormonal abnormalities have been identified. Hormonal agents which improve mastalgia act at different sites on the hypothalamic-pituitary-ovarian-breast axis and this makes it likely that the aetiology of mastalgia is either multifactorial or that the final common pathway is at the breast cell level.

Water retention within the breast has been suggested as a cause of both mastalgia and the premenstrual tension syndrome because women report weight gain and breast and ankle swelling late in the menstrual cycle. Studies have shown that patients with mastalgia do not retain more water than women without this symptom. This information combined with the finding that diuretics are no more effective in mastalgia than placebo suggests that water retention is unlikely to be the cause of cyclical mastalgia.

A theory prevalent some years ago was that patients with mastalgia were more neurotic than other patients and that this manifested itself as a complaint of breast pain. This has now been shown to have little scientific foundation.

The role of essential fatty acids (EFAs)

The chance finding that there was a reduction in breast pain in women treated with evening primrose oil (EPO), which contains high levels of gamma linolenic acid (GLA), led to the investigation of the role of GLA and other EFAs in patients with mastalgia. EFAs must be provided regularly in the diet and have three major functions:

1. They are key determinants of cellular membrane flexibility and fluidity.

   In cellular membranes, EFAs are present as either free fatty acids, triglycerides or are esterified to phospholipids and cholesterol. They compete with saturated fatty acids for incorporation into these membranes. EFAs confer the properties of flexibility and fluidity to membranes and thereby affect the activity of membrane-bound receptors. Hormone receptors, present within cellular membranes rich in saturated fatty acids, have a greater affinity for their respective hormones than those receptors found in membranes rich in polyunsaturated fatty acids. Therefore in an environment with a high saturated to polyunsaturated fatty acid ratio, increased receptor affinity and hormone potency will result in an exaggerated end organ response to normal circulating hormone levels.

2. They are precursors of biologically active metabolites.

The metabolites of GLA are precursors of a wide range of short-lived biologically active molecules, which regulate many aspects of cellular activity, collectively known as the eicosanoids; prostaglandins, leukotrienes and other derivatives are produced locally as and when required and have a purely local effect after which they are eliminated. Prostaglandin E_1 (PGE_1), which is produced from EFAs, is known to be a second messenger for prolactin and, as prolactin levels rise, PGE_1 formation increases to switch off the peripheral effect of prolactin. Low levels of GLA and its metabolites may therefore result in a reduction in the levels of PGE_1 and lead to an exaggerated end organ response to prolactin.

The effects of GLA on membrane receptors and on eicosanoid and prostaglandin production might explain why normal levels of hormones produce exaggerated effects such as severe mastalgia.

3. EFAs have a role in the transport of cholesterol.

Cholesterol is transported to cells in low density lipoproteins (LDLs) and from cells to the liver in high density lipoproteins (HDLs). Women with mastalgia have been reported to have high levels of HDLs and low levels of LDLs in the absence of a difference in dietary fat intake.

Interestingly, hormonal drug treatments which improve symptoms of mastalgia influence plasma lipids, generally by producing a reduction in HDLs. The effect of GLA on plasma lipids is poorly described but it has been reported to reduce total cholesterol and to have variable effects on HDLs and LDLs. In view of the action of the recognized treatments for mastalgia on lipid metabolism, it is possible that the underlying aetiology of patients with mastalgia could be an abnormality in lipid metabolism.

Women with mastalgia have been found to have abnormal plasma fatty acid profiles. Treatment with GLA in the form of Efamast, eight capsules (320 mg GLA) daily for 4 months produces a progressive increase towards normal fatty acid profiles. Following a period of treatment, fatty acid profiles fall back to pretreatment levels and this is consistent with observations from clinical studies where mastalgia recurs in up to half of patients who gain a beneficial response to GLA.

Assessment

The first and most important consideration is to exclude any underlying specific cause for the pain. The cyclical nature of the pain and the effects of any treatment are best assessed using pain charts completed each day by the patient (Fig. 3.2). Reassurance has long been recognized as the most important part of the management and, as long ago as 1879, Bilroth wrote that 'friendly advice, reassurance and the banishment and suspicion and fear of dread disease is of great importance'. This involves taking a careful history and performing a full examination of the breast and, if considered appropriate, mammography and/or ultrasound. If a dominant or discrete lump is present, management is as for any other mass lesion; likewise if there is any suspicious lesion visible on mammography this requires appropriate investigation. Thereafter it has been demonstrated that reassurance alone is sufficient for over 85% of patients.

Drugs used in the treatment of mastalgia

Diuretics

There is no scientific rationale for prescribing diuretics for cyclical mastalgia. Double-blind, placebo-controlled studies have shown no benefit and these drugs no longer have a place in the management of cyclical breast pain.

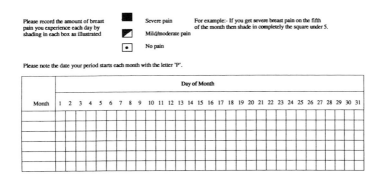

Fig. 3.2 Example of a pain chart. This allows a visual assessment of the severity and extent of pain.

Vitamin B6 — pyridoxine

This has been shown to be of some benefit in patients with the premenstrual syndrome. It is possibly of benefit in relief of mild tenderness but in randomized, controlled trials has not caused significant improvements, and it is therefore no longer considered an appropriate treatment for breast pain.

Danazol

Danazol is a synthetic steroid with anti-gonadotrophic properties. Its action in humans has not been clearly defined. Although it can inhibit the secretion of luteinizing hormone and follicle-stimulating hormone, it only does so in the human in very high dosage. It has a local tissue effect and has been shown to bind to both progesterone and androgen receptors but not to oestrogen receptors. Controlled, double-blind, randomized trials have clearly shown that danazol is beneficial in cyclical mastalgia producing both relief of symptoms and reduction in nodularity at doses as low as 200 mg. It is the most effective agent for severe breast pain and produces improvement in approximately 70% of patients (Table 3.2).

The main problem with danazol is its side-effect profile (Table 3.3). There has been a high drop out rate in studies because of these side-effects which include a 5% lowering of voice pitch. This has been permanent in a small number of patients. Other side-effects include hirsuitism and weight gain.

Once a patient's pain is under control with a dose of 200 mg daily, then it is usually possible to reduce patients to a maintenance dose of 100 mg daily on alternate days.

GLA

The fatty acid deficiency hypothesis has led to the testing of treatment by supplementing the diet with the EFA GLA. EPO is a natural source of GLA which is prescribed as Efamast. It has proved

Table 3.2 Response of drug treatment in cyclical and non-cyclical mastalgia

| | % useful response | | |
	Cyclical	Non-cyclical	% side-effects
Danazol	79	40	30
GLA	58	38	4
Bromocriptine	54	33	35

Table 3.3 Drawbacks and side-effects of drugs to treat mastalgia

---

Gamolenic acid
- Mild nausea
- Slow response to treatment

Danazol
- Weight gain
- Acne
- Hirsuitism

Bromocriptine
- Nausea
- Dizziness

---

useful in mild to moderate cyclical mastalgia and, importantly, it has virtually no side-effects (Table 3.3). Patient acceptance is high as it is viewed as a natural substance rather than a hormone or a drug. A useful response is obtained in approximately 60% of patients (Table 3.2). The dose is 6–8 capsules per day.

Bromocriptine

This drug reduces prolactin levels and has proved consistently effective in relieving cyclical mastalgia. It is at least as effective as GLA, although it has a much higher incidence of side-effects. Dosage is 2.5 mg twice daily which is introduced slowly increasing the dose over 1–2 weeks. The major problem with bromocriptine is that over 30% of women experience side-effects and in 20% these are severe (Table 3.3). These side-effects are reduced by introducing the drug slowly and avoiding a dosage higher than 5 mg/day. A newer anti-prolactin agent, cabergoline, is now available. It is given in a dose of 500 mcg once weekly. Its effectiveness in breast pain is currently being assessed in clinical trials.

Tamoxifen

At present tamoxifen does not have a product licence for use in breast pain. A small number of studies have assessed its effectiveness in cyclical breast pain and in one small study 71% of patients achieved a reduction in their breast pain when treated with a dose of 20 mg. Side-effects were reported by 26%, the most common complaints being hot flushes and increased vaginal discharge.

Luteinizing hormone releasing hormone (LHRH) analogues

Although this may be effective in over 90% of patients with cyclical mastalgia, unacceptable side-effects follow this treatment and include hot flushes in 87%, headache in 57%, diminished libido in 37%, nausea or vomiting in 28% and depression/irritability in 24%. This drug cannot therefore be recommended for routine use in patients with cyclical breast pain. The preparations currently available are also very expensive.

Management of patients with moderate and severe mastalgia in primary care

Patients with minor and moderate degrees of breast pain who do not have a discrete palpable lesion can be managed initially by their general practitioner. Having ascertained that the pain is cyclical, that it lasts more than 7 days a month and is interfering with life, these patients should be treated initially with gamolenic acid as in Figure 3.3. Patients should be treated with gamolenic acid for an initial period of at least 4 months. After 4 months of treatment, if there is no response to GLA, then it is appropriate either to refer the patient to hospital for further management or to change to danazol (200–300 mg daily, slowly reduced to 100 mg a day after relief of symptoms) or to bromocriptine (2.5 mg twice daily introduced gradually by increasing this dose over 1–2 weeks). Both drugs should be used only by patients who are not taking oral contraceptives and are using adequate mechanical contraception. As outlined above, side-effects are more common with these drugs. The side-effects and cost of danazol treatment can be limited by reducing the dose. Response may be maintained by doses as low as 100 mg on alternate days or 100 mg daily given on days 14–28 of the menstrual cycle (Fig. 3.4).

For patients with very severe mastalgia, the agent of first choice is danazol. Patients with severe pain should be seen and assessed in hospital and drugs such as tamoxifen or LHRH agonists should only be prescribed through hospitals as these drugs are not currently licensed for breast pain in the UK.

Surgery

A small number of patients who have cyclical breast pain either fail to respond to any treatment or relapse following successive courses of different agents. Some of these patients are improved by bilateral mastectomy and breast reconstruction. Such patients require

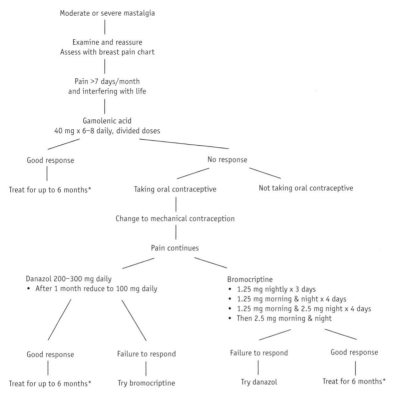

Fig. 3.3   Protocol for treating moderate to severe cyclical mastalgia (mild mastalgia requires examination and reassurance). ★ After 6 months treatment should be stopped. Breast pain will recur in only 50% of patients, and some of these will not need further treatment because the pain is milder. Severe recurrences can be treated with a further course of previously successful treatment.

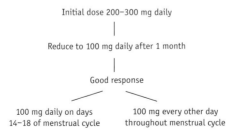

Fig. 3.4   Protocol for reducing dosage of danazol.

very careful assessment, often with the help of a psychologist. It is clear that some of those patients who have undergone this operation continue to complain of pain and the current view is that this operation is rarely indicated.

Natural history of cyclical mastalgia

Cyclical pain is often relieved by pregnancy and the menopause. Patients with cyclical pain who start having symptoms at an early age tend to have persistent pain throughout their reproductive life whereas patients who have a late age of onset have a shorter overall duration of pain. Treatment in young patients often, therefore, has to be for prolonged periods. The current aim is to treat young patients with severe mastalgia with short, intermittent bursts rather than continuous periods. Many patients with mastalgia do get spontaneous remission of their symptoms.

Other measures

Some patients appear to benefit from wearing a well-fitting brassiere worn 24 h/day. Between 5% and 15% of patients have pain of such a degree they require specific treatment. Reduction of caffeine intake and a low fat diet have been suggested to be effective in mastalgia, but few studies have scientifically evaluated these measures. Regular exercise has been reported to improve breast pain. Soya, which has a high content of phyto-oestrogens is currently being evaluated in breast pain.

Summary of management of patients with cyclical mastalgia

- Exclude cancer.
- Reassure and check for properly fitting bra.
- Define pattern of pain — pain charts.
- Drug treatment
    first line GLA
    second line danazol
    third line bromocriptine
    fourth line tamoxifen and/or LHRH agonists (useful if pain
      is severe and not responding rapidly to other agents).

NON-CYCLICAL MASTALGIA

Non-cyclical mastalgia is breast pain with a time pattern which is not associated with cyclical ovarian function. It may be continuous but usually has a random time pattern. Non-cyclical mastalgia is associated with a wide range of apparently unrelated events and conditions. These are usually local rather than systemic, that is their cause is located either in the breast or chest wall. Non-cyclical mastalgia arises either because of localized pain in the chest wall, referred pain, or diffuse true breast pain and these three types of breast pain must be differentiated (Table 3.4). Appropriate treatment should be started for referred pain. Chest wall causes of breast pain include Tietze syndrome where one or more costal cartridge posterior to the breast is enlarged, painful and tender. Patients can also present with localized pain in the lateral chest wall arising from underlying muscles. In these patients, the breast can be lifted away from the chest wall without discomfort, whereas deep palpation produces severe pain. Up to 60% of patients with a persistent localized painful area in the chest wall can be effectively treated by infiltration with local anaesthetic and steroid (2 ml of 1% lignocaine combined with 40 mg of methylprednisolone in 1 ml). Production of a pain-free area by injection of local anaesthetic confirms the diagnosis. There is some recent evidence that application of non-steroidal gels directly over the area of tenderness improves localized chest wall pain.

Particular benign breast disorders are strongly associated with non-cyclical mastalgia and these include periductal mastitis, fat necrosis and sclerosing adenosis. Some women have a localized single area of tenderness in the breast which is known as a trigger spot. Some of these respond to injection of local anaesthetic and steroid. It has been reported that pain can be eliminated in up to half of these women by excision of the trigger spot. However, surgery generally makes breast pain worse — some women develop non-cyclical breast pain at the site of previous breast operations.

Table 3.4 Classification of non-cyclical mastalgia

Chest wall causes
- For example, tender costochondral junctions (Tietze syndrome)

True breast pain
- Diffuse breast pain
- Trigger spots in breast

Non-breast causes
- Cervical and thoracic spondylosis
- Bornholm disease
- Lung disease
- Gallstones
- Exogenous oestrogens such as hormone replacement therapy
- Thoracic outlet syndrome

Excision of tender painful areas in an attempt to relieve symptoms is therefore rarely appropriate. For patients with true breast pain, wearing a firm supporting bra 24 h a day often improves this pain. True diffuse pain should be treated initially with non-steroidal anti-inflammatory drugs. If this fails, some women respond to drugs used for cyclical mastalgia. Because of its low incidence of side-effects, GLA should be the first of these agents to be tried.

Treatment of non-cyclical mastalgia

- Exclude specific causes such as Tietze syndrome and musculo-skeletal influences.
- Wear a firm supporting bra 24 h/day.
- Simple analgesia.
- Less than 40% respond to hormonal agents (Table 3.2) — GLA should be the first of these agents tried because of its low incidence of side-effects.

    If there is a persistent localized painful area then the use of local anaesthetic and steroid injection is effective in the short term in up to 70% of sufferers.

    A non-steroidal anti-inflammatory agent may be useful for the group with musculoskeletal pain.

NODULARITY

Nodularity in the breast may be diffuse or focal. As previously noted premenstrual nodularity is such a common finding that it should be considered normal. Generalized nodularity was previously considered to be abnormal and termed fibroadenosis and fibrocystic disease. This is unfortunate since it is now clear that there is little correlation between generalized nodularity and the underlying histological appearances. These terms are, therefore, inappropriate and should no longer be used.

GENERALIZED NODULARITY

Breasts are normally nodular and, in almost all instances, generalized nodularity is normal.

Management

- Clinical examination.
- Mammography if over 35 years.
- Reassure if no clinical or mammographic abnormality.

In the absence of any clinical or radiological abnormality, these patients require reassurance that their breasts are normal and that, as a group, they are no more likely to develop breast cancer than women whose breasts do not have generalized nodularity.

FOCAL NODULARITY

Incidence

This is the most common cause of a breast lump up to the age of 50. Although accounting for up to 70% of breast lumps in women under the age of 40, localized benign nodularity remains a very common cause of a breast lump until after the menopause. Although within an area of localized nodularity there can be areas of localized fibrosis, an increase in the number of glandular elements (adenosis), the presence of small cysts and areas of apocrine change — all these changes are now considered part of normal breast involution; they are also often present in other areas of the same breast which are not nodular and are a common finding in the normal population of women of this age. Localized nodularity is only rarely associated with a focal pathological abnormality such as a localized area of sclerosis, epithelial hyperplasia or a breast cancer.

Management

- Clinical examination.
- Mammography if over 35 years.
- Ultrasound is often of use.
- FNAC if discrete area.
- Biopsy indicated if clinical, cytological or radiological suspicion of malignancy.

Some units biopsy all patients with localized nodularity over the age of 40 who do not have definitive evidence that the lesion is benign — that is those patients who do not have completely lucent mammograms or one or even two FNAC reports which show benign elements only. These women should be reassured and discharged if appropriate investigations show no abnormality. They do not require regular follow up as, in some women, this increases anxiety.

DISORDERS OF INVOLUTION

Breast involution is usually obvious by the age of 35. The changes include the disappearance of lobular epithelium and specialized lobular connective tissue, with replacement by the more usual fibrous tissue found in the interlobular region. Aberrations of breast involution include macrocyst formation, sclerosis and failure of all breast tissue to involute at the same rate. During involution there can be an increase in the number of cells lining the terminal duct lobular unit — epithelial hyperplasia.

CYSTIC DISEASE OF THE BREAST

Cystic disease of the breast is a term which should be restricted to the clearly defined group of women who present with palpable breast cysts. Terms such as fibrocystic disease and cystic mastopathy should no longer be in clinical use.

Astley Cooper in 1829 first distinguished cysts as separate entities from breast cancer. In the early 1900s, workers postulated that cysts arose as a consequence of senile involution of breast lobules and this remains the currently held view of their pathogenesis.

Incidence

Approximately 7% of all women in the western world present at some time during their life to hospital with a palpable breast cyst.

Cysts are most common in the perimenopausal age group and they are uncommon after the menopause (Fig. 2.17, see page 29).

Aetiology of cystic disease

There is considerable indirect evidence that cystic disease is hormonally related — its bilateral nature, its relationship to the menopause and the response of cystic disease to endocrine treatment. There is no convincing direct evidence, however, that women who develop breast cysts have a different profile of plasma hormones to those without cysts. Studies have shown that the levels of EFAs in the plasma of patients with cysts are lower than in the general population.

Clinical aspects of cystic disease

Presentation

The majority of patients present with a smooth discrete breast lump which may be fluctuant. Non-fluctuant, so called 'tension cysts', can clinically resemble a carcinoma. Pain can be a presenting symptom (less than 30%) and cysts can also be discovered incidentally during the screening process. The total number of palpable breast cysts a woman develops varies greatly between individuals; approximately one-half develop only a single cyst, one-third have between two and five cysts and the remainder more than five. Cysts are more common in the left than right breast, as is breast cancer. About one-third of patients have cysts in both breasts.

Management

All patients over 35 years should have a mammogram prior to needle aspiration as 1–3% of patients with cysts have an incidental carcinoma (Fig. 3.5).

- Aspirate with a 21g needle.
- If multiple cysts are present, ultrasound is as specific as aspiration in determining whether the lesions are cystic.
- If fluid is obtained, aspirate cyst to dryness.
- No fluid to cytology unless evenly bloodstained.
- Examine patient after aspiration to determine if residual mass. If mass present requires investigation with cytology, ultrasound and/or biopsy.
- Review patient 3–6 weeks after cyst aspiration to check for refilling. Cysts which rapidly or persistently refill more than twice should be excised as there is an association between repeated and rapid refilling and malignancy.

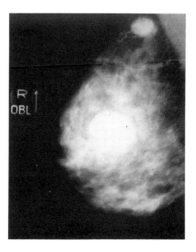

Fig. 3.5 Mammogram of a breast cyst. There is an incidental breast cancer which was not initially suspected on clinical examination.

Risk of carcinoma

Patients who develop breast cysts are at some increased risk (relative risk 1.5–4 times) of developing breast carcinoma (Table 3.5). The risk is greatest in young patients (<45) where the relative risk may be as high as six times that of the general population. Debate continues on whether these young women should have earlier and more regular screening than is currently available through the government screening programme.

Treatment of patients with multiple cysts

In the majority of patients with multiple cysts no treatment is indicated. In particular these women should not be subjected to regular aspiration of asymptomatic cysts. These patients can be assessed by regular ultrasound and mammographic assessment of their breasts performed every 1–2 years. Only symptomatic cysts require aspiration.

SCLEROSIS

Sclerosing adenosis, radial scars and complex sclerosing lesions (this term incorporates the lesions previously called sclerosing papillomatosis or duct adenoma and includes infiltrating epitheliosis) are all examples of sclerosis occurring in the period of breast involution. These lesions are important because they can cause diagnostic problems to the surgeon, radiologist and pathologist (Fig. 3.6). Sclerosing adenosis and radial scars are both associated with distortion of the terminal duct lobular unit and yet show no significant hyperplasia.

Table 3.5 Incidence of breast cancer in women with breast cysts

Author	Year	No of women	Follow-up (years)	No of cancers	Relative risk
Chardot	1970	206	5	6	7.5
Haagensen	1984	2511	5–30	72	2.48
Roberts et al	1984	428	10–15	17	3.5
Jones & Bradbeer	1980	332	5	7	2.5
Harrington & Lesnick	1980	596	5.6	19	3.5
Bundred et al	1991	352	5–12	14	4.4
Ciatto et al	1990	3809	1–7	34	1.77
Bruzzi et al	1997	802	6	17	4.24
Dixon et al	1997	1374	9	65	3.25

The first three studies listed include patients with cystic disease diagnosed by both biopsy and aspiration, whereas the remaining studies include patients diagnosed by aspiration alone

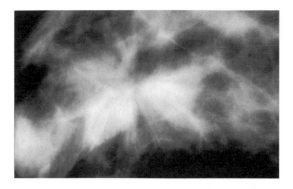

Fig. 3.6 Mammogram of a radial scar. Some are similar in appearance to tubular carcinomas.

Complex sclerosing lesions which are less common are more frequently associated with significant degrees of epithelial hyperplasia.

There is some debate as to whether radial scars might be the precursors of invasive tubular carcinomas although the current view is that these lesions should not be considered premalignant or a significant risk factor for subsequent breast cancer. Areas of sclerosis are best considered aberrations of breast involution and, following excision, follow up is not required unless the lesion is associated with significant degrees of epithelial hyperplasia.

Clinical features

Patients with these conditions may either present with a breast lump or breast pain, or have an asymptomatic mammographic abnormality detected at a centre which has a screening programme. In such instances they are usually impalpable.

Management

FNAC performed free hand if the lesion is palpable, or stereotactically if impalpable, often indicates that the lesion is benign.

Excisional biopsy is often required to make a definitive diagnosis.

EPITHELIAL HYPERPLASIA

An increase in the number of layers of epithelial cells lining the terminal duct lobular unit is known as epithelial hyperplasia. Previously this change was called epitheliosis or papillomatosis but these terms can now be regarded as obsolete. The degree of hyperplasia can be graded as mild, moderate or florid. Mild hyperplasia, which is more than two but not more than four epithelial cells in depth, is associated with no greater risk of invasive breast carcinoma than comparable women who do not have this feature.

Clinical significance of epithelial hyperplasia

Patients with moderate and florid degrees of epithelial hyperplasia but which do not have atypical features (proliferative disease without atypia) are considered to have a slightly increased (1.5–2 times) risk of invasive carcinoma relative to comparable women who do not have this feature. Women who have a lesion which shows a combination of hyperplasia and cellular atypia, known as atypical hyperplasia, have a risk of developing breast cancer 4–5 times that of the general population and are at moderately increased risk. It is only this order of risk which is considered significant. There is a strong interaction with family history and atypical hyperplasia, and it is relevant to consider women with atypical hyperplasia who have a positive family history separately from those who do not. A definition of a positive family history is that at least one first-degree relative — be it mother, daughter, sister — has proven breast cancer.

The clinical significance of epithelial hyperplasia can be best appreciated by the analysis of the proportion of patients with the various lesions who have developed breast cancer during a prolonged follow-up period. This analysis is shown in Figure 3.7 and demonstrates that the absolute risk of breast cancer development in a women with atypical hyperplasia without a family history is 8% at 10 years, whereas in those with a positive family history the risk is 20–25% at 15 years. The magnitude of risk for women with atypical hyperplasia and a positive family history is very similar to that for certain types of carcinoma *in situ*.

Clinical features

Patients with atypical hyperplasia do not present with typical clinical signs which allow a clinical diagnosis to be made. They can present with a lump, lumpiness, nipple discharge or be identified as having either a localized clinical or mammographic abnormality detected by screening. When a fine needle aspirate is performed from an area of moderate or florid hyperplasia, with or without atypia, the aspirate is usually markedly cellular and in some instances the cells show atypical features. These lesions are, there-

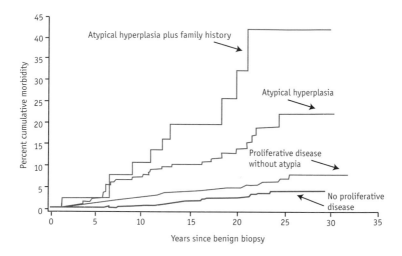

Fig. 3.7 Percentage of patients developing breast cancer after a biopsy showing atypical hyperplasia with or without family history.

fore, usually reported as suspicious or highly suspicious of malignancy on FNAC. Mammographically, areas of hyperplasia may be associated with areas of distortion of architecture, as in a complex sclerosing lesion, or they can be associated with microcalcification and are diagnosed only after a localization biopsy. The majority of epithelial hyperplasias are, however, not associated with any specific symptoms.

Management

- Moderate and florid hyperplasia: no clinically significant risk and therefore no further follow up required.
- Atypical hyperplasia: determine whether there is a positive family history so the absolute risk can be estimated and discussed with the patient. Options are close clinical and mammographic surveillance, entry into prevention studies or mastectomy (total or subcutaneous) with immediate reconstruction.

RESIDUAL BREAST TISSUE

In some individuals not all breast tissue involutes at the same rate and therefore results in clinical and mammographic asymmetry, and this can sometimes be difficult to differentiate from breast cancer.

Management

FNAC and mammography repeated after an interval of 3–6 months are the best methods of establishing whether an area of clinical nodularity or localized mammographic density are due to this condition.

GYNAECOMASTIA

Growth of breast tissue in males to any extent at all ages is known as gynaecomastia. It is an entirely benign condition and usually reversible. The degree of enlargement varies and, in extreme cases, the size or shape may be similar to that of the female breast. Histologically the changes are identical to those described in virginal hypertrophy.

Age incidence

Gynaecomastia occurs in three different age groups. The first is found in the neonatal period in which palpable breast tissue transiently develops in 6–90% of all new-born babies because of transplacental passage of oestrogens. Puberty and old age are the other times when gynaecomastia commonly occurs.

Pubertal gynaecomastia

This affects boys between the ages of 10 and 19, with the peak incidence being between the ages of 13 and 14. Some degree of pubertal gynaecomastia occurs in between 30% and 70% of boys if carefully sought. The aetiology and hormonal basis are not completely understood although it is probably due to an oestrogen/androgen imbalance. It usually requires no treatment as 80% spontaneously resolve within 2 years. Occasionally, because it is unsightly and embarrassing, subcutaneous mastectomy is indicated. This operation can usually be performed through a small circumareolar incision. During the operation a small disk of breast tissue should be left attached to the undersurface of the areola and some fat should remain on the skin flaps to ensure that the end result is not an unsightly depression in the anterior chest wall. Alternatives to excisional surgery include liposuction using a dissecting cannula. Patient dissatisfaction with the end result of surgery is common and the possibility of a less than perfect result must be explicitly discussed with the patient.

Adult gynaecomastia

Senescent gynaecomastia commonly affects males aged between 50 and 80 years. In the majority it does not appear to be associated with any endocrine abnormality although there may be an underlying luteinizing hormone/follicle stimulating hormone imbalance.

Specific causes of gynaecomastia need to be considered and include drugs, cirrhosis, malnutrition, hypogonadism and testicular tumours. The relative frequency of these different causes is outlined in Table 3.6.

Clinical features of gynaecomastia

Breast lesions are usually soft, involve the whole gland and are commonly bilateral. Unilateral eccentric, tender, hard or ulcerating lesions suggest the underlying pathology may be breast cancer. In these cases mammography is often useful and FNAC will usually indicate if the mass is malignant.

Indications for investigation

Gynaecomastia is common and the finding of non-tender palpable breast tissue on routine examination does not require any evaluation. In most instances a careful history is sufficient to uncover most of the conditions associated with gynaecomastia. If no abnormalities are found on physical examination to explain the gynaecomastia the patient should be re-examined again in 6 months.

A history of recent onset of progressive breast enlargement, with or without pain and tenderness, without an easily identifiable cause (such as an underlying disease or specific drug therapy) is an indication for investigation. In such instances blood should be taken to assess liver, renal and thyroid function. If no clear cause is apparent when the results of these investigations are available then blood hormone levels should be measured to exclude a hormone-producing tumour.

Table 3.6 Causes of gynaecomastia expressed as a percentage

Cause	%
Puberty	25
Idiopathic (senescent)	25
Drugs (cimetidine, digoxin, spironolactone, androgens or anti-oestrogens)	10–20
Cirrhosis or malnutrition	8
Primary hypogonadism	8
Testicular tumours	3
Secondary hypogonadism	2
Hyperthyroidism	1.5
Renal disease	1

FAT NECROSIS

Fat necrosis of the breast was first described as a clinical entity in 1920. It accounts for approximately one in 200 of all breast problems.

Aetiology and pathogenesis

Fat necrosis was originally thought to be secondary to trauma and it is often called 'traumatic fat necrosis'. In fact a history of trauma is present in less than 40% of patients. Nowadays it is often seen after road traffic accidents as a result of seat belt trauma to the breast (Fig. 3.8).

Clinical features

Fat necrosis is of clinical concern because it is sometimes difficult to distinguish from carcinoma on both physical examination and mammography. Characteristically there is a painless mass in the breast which is firm, ill defined and poorly mobile. Associated skin thickening or retraction are often seen and this increases the clinical suspicion that the lesion may be malignant. It can occur anywhere in the breast but it is most common in the subareolar region. Following resolution fat cysts may remain in the breast.

Management

- If there is a definite history of trauma and overlying bruising and a palpable mass is present, then management should be initially by observation.
- It is important to note there may be an initial increase in size of the mass.
- FNAC ± core biopsy and mammography should be performed.
- If suspicion of malignancy persists a biopsy is indicated.

BREAST HAEMATOMA

Haematoma is the most common breast problem following trauma. This may be major trauma following a road traffic accident or local trauma from an aspirate or fine needle aspirate, core needle or open biopsy. The mammographic appearance of a haematoma may be ominous with poorly defined margins raising the possibility of a carcinoma. Because it is known that haematomas can follow FNAC, and that these may mimic cancer, it is now practice to perform mammography prior to FNAC.

In extremely unusual circumstances breast carcinoma may present with spontaneous haemorrhage and a haematoma in the absence of breast trauma. Ultrasound can be useful in the diagnosis of a breast haematoma.

Breast haematoma may also occur spontaneously in patients on anticoagulant therapy.

Management

- Small haematomas following direct trauma or needle aspiration are treated with support, analgesia and observation.
- Large haematomas occurring spontaneously with evidence of overlying skin thinning or following surgery may need formal drainage.

It is important to appreciate that some patients with breast cancer present with a recent history of trauma. Failure of a haematoma to resolve rapidly, particularly after a fine needle aspirate which has failed to provide diagnostic information, is an indication for open biopsy.

GALACTOCELE

This is a cystic lesion occurring in women during or after pregnancy or breast feeding. It contains breast milk which may be inspissated. It is said to be more frequent in women who stop breast feeding suddenly. Treatment is by aspiration which both confirms the diagnosis and usually cures the condition.

BLOCKED MONTGOMERY'S TUBERCULES

These glands on the surface of the areola can become obstructed and the sebaceous secretion builds up and presents as a periareolar lump which, if troublesome, can be excised.

BENIGN NEOPLASMS

Duct papilloma

These lesions can be single or multiple. They are very common and, because of their frequency, it has been suggested that they might best be considered as aberrations rather than true benign neoplasms. They show minimal if any malignant potential. There is some debate as to whether patients with the so-called 'multiple papilloma syndrome' are at increased risk of subsequent breast cancer although this is disputed.

Symptoms

The most frequent symptom is spontaneous nipple discharge which can be serous or bloodstained. Even serous discharges from patients with a duct papilloma are usually positive for blood on 'stix testing. Occasionally in large papillomas the patients also present with a breast mass.

Clinical features

Characteristically the discharge emanates from a single duct. As there is often duct dilatation distal to the papilloma, pressure over the dilated duct at the areola margin produces large amounts of discharge. The discharge itself is usually either bloodstained or is positive for blood on testing. Occasionally a palpable mass is present at the areola margin which can represent either the papilloma itself or the dilated duct beyond.

Management

- Perform mammography.
- Test for blood.
- Discuss possibility of ductogram with radiologist.
- If positive for blood or the discharge is persistent or troublesome, the patient may require excision of the involved duct.

Treatment

Excision of a duct or 'microdochectomy' can be performed through a very small circumareolar incision. As the majority of causes of duct discharge occur within the first 2 cm of the major subareolar duct it is usually only necessary to excise a small portion of the diseased duct.

LIPOMAS

Lipomas are common both within the subcutaneous tissue over the breast and within the breast. The main interest in this lesion lies in the confusion with a 'pseudolipoma' which is a soft mass which can be felt around a small breast cancer caused by indrawing of the fat by a spiculated carcinoma.

Clinical presentation

Patients present with a soft lobulated, localized mass in the subcutaneous tissue or within the breast itself.

Management

- Establish diagnosis by mammography/FNAC.
- Excise only if suspicion of malignancy or if troublesome.

COSMETIC SURGERY

Breast augmentation

Indications

Although these include breast asymmetry resulting from congenital anomalies, the main reason for patients requesting breast augmentation is a desire to increase the size of their breasts. There are few operations in which it is more difficult to evaluate the outcome. The operation itself produces a remarkable degree of happiness and there is almost uniform improvement in self image. Only 1% of women who have had this operation performed say that they are unhappy with the result and would not have it performed again.

Technique

Most patients can be adequately treated by insertion of a prosthesis usually placed under the breast tissue itself or under the pectoralis major muscle. For patients who have small truncated breasts which lack tissue in all dimensions (known as tuberous or tubular breasts), it is often necessary to insert a tissue expander initially and then replace this with a permanent prosthesis.

Prostheses and their problems

A variety of materials have been used to increase the size of the breast. These include silicone implants, saline-filled prostheses and a combination of both. Saline-filled prostheses are associated with a high rate of saline leakage (more than 15%) with subsequent spontaneous deflation and this has thrown these into disfavour. Double lumen prostheses are difficult to fabricate and have many potential problems. Currently the best cosmetic results are obtained with a silicone gel-filled prosthesis. There is no evidence, clinical or otherwise, of carcinogenesis resulting from their use. At present there is no conclusive proof that they cause autoimmune disease, but the increasing number of anecdotal reports of connective tissue disease in women who have been the recipients of such implants merits further investigation. A prospective registration programme for patients undergoing augmentation has been introduced to try and resolve this problem. A newer prosthesis filled with soya oil (but still enclosed in a silicone shell) is being marketed on the premise that any leakage will not cause problems. These have only been on the market for a short while and their long-term efficacy is, as yet, unknown.

Postoperative technical and mechanical problems, such as implant deflation, perforation, rupture, creasing or palpable folds, may occasionally be encountered. Other complications of such surgery include capsular contracture and, rarely, infection. These complications may require surgical revision and removal or exchange of the implant but do not in themselves make breast implants dangerous. The consensus view is that silicone breast implants are safe.

The most common postoperative complication of augmentation and reconstructive mammoplasty using silicone prostheses is the formation of, and subsequent contraction of, fibrous capsules around implants. Capsule formation around an implant is universal and has been reported with all types, shapes, surfaces and sizes of prostheses. The reported incidence of clinically significant capsular contracture ranges from 3–74%. This variation reflects different methods of measurement. It appears to occur less commonly with saline-filled than gel-filled implants. There is some evidence that textured implants which have an irregular surface reduce contracture rates; in one study they decreased the incidence of capsular contracture at 1 year from 58% to 8%. The majority of implants used in the UK at the present time are, therefore, textured silicone gel-filled prostheses.

Much publicity has surrounded the 'bleed' of silicone gel from the prosthesis. It has been known for some time that minute amounts of silicone gel leak or bleed through the envelope of prostheses and can migrate to other organs. There is no evidence that the silicone gel bleed is either responsible for the capsule formation or causes problems when it migrates to other organs.

Reduction mammoplasty

Indications

The reasons for performing reduction mammoplasty include juvenile hypertrophy, generally large breasts and achievement of symmetry in patients with asymmetrical breasts resulting from either congenital anomalies or surgery. One common indication for reduction mammoplasty is to reduce the size of one breast to match the size of a contralateral reconstructed breast following mastectomy for breast cancer. Patients need to be informed of the scars that will result from this surgery and possible complications.

The complications that follow this type of surgery relate to wound healing, scarring, infection and haematoma formation.

Technique

Breast reduction is accomplished by maintaining the nipple and areola on a pedicle of breast tissue and re-siting it after excision of skin and breast tissue. The new site for the nipple/areola complex is carefully marked prior to operation (Fig. 3.9). The skin is then mobilized from the underlying breast tissue and the bulk of breast reduced either circumferentially around or inferiorly to the nipple/areola pedicle. Scars resulting from this procedure leave an inverted T pattern.

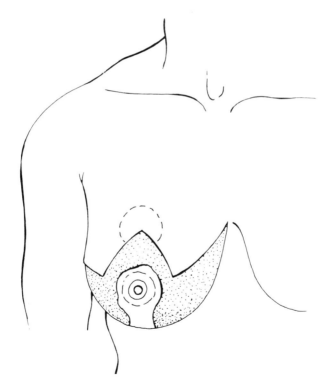

Fig. 3.9 Lines of incision for reduction mammoplasty using an inferior dermal flap technique; the dotted line represents the ideal new position of the nipple.

Mastopexy ('breast lift')

Ptosis (sagging) of the breast is common following pregnancy. Mastopexy is indicated where there is severe ptosis and is commonly called 'a breast lift'.

Technique

Simple nipple/areola advancement will help but usually some skin excision either by removal of a V-shaped portion of skin inferiorly, or an excision of skin (as in reduction mammoplasty) are required. A mastopexy can be combined with an augmentation to fill out the loose skin and replace some of the breast tissue which has disappeared.

4. Breast infection

INTRODUCTION

Breast infection is much less common than it used to be. It is seen occasionally in neonates but most commonly affects adult females between the ages of 18 and 50. In the adult, breast infection can be considered as lactational or non-lactational. Infection can also affect the skin overlying the breast and can occur either as a primary event or secondary to a lesion within the skin such as a sebaceous cyst or to an underlying condition such as hidradenitis suppurativa. The organisms responsible for different types of breast infection, and the most appropriate antibiotics for treating these organisms, are summarized in Table 4.1. The guiding principles in treating breast infection are:

- Antibiotics should be given early to abort abscess formation.
- Hospital referral is indicated if the infection does not settle rapidly with antibiotics.
- If an abscess is suspected this should be confirmed by aspiration.

Table 4.1 Organisms responsible for different types of breast infection and appropriate antibiotics

| Type of infection | Organism | Antibiotic | |
		No penicillin allergy	Penicillin allergy
Neonatal Lactating Skin associated	*Staph. aureus*	Flucloxacillin	Erythromycin
Non-lactating	*Staph. aureus* Enterococci Anaerobic Streptococci *Bacteroides species*	Augmentin	Combination of cephradine or erythromycin and metronidazole

- If the lesion is solid on aspiration then a sample of cells should be obtained for cytology to exclude an underlying inflammatory carcinoma.
  Specific infections affecting the breast can be defined.

MASTITIS NEONATORUM

Aetiology and pathogenesis

Continued enlargement of the breast bud in the first week or two of life occurs in about 60% of new-born babies and the gland may reach several centimetres in size before regressing. Although *Staphylococcus aureus* (*Staph. aureus*) is the usual organism, *Escherichia coli* (*E. coli*) can sometimes cause this infection.

Clinical features

Neonatal breast buds are usually red and somewhat tender but infection is uncommon. When infection is present the breast bud becomes hard, tender and erythematous. Abscess formation can follow and some infants become severely ill.

Management

If an abscess develops, incision and drainage should be performed under general anaesthetic and combined with intravenous antibiotics. The incision should be made as peripherally as possible.

LACTATING BREAST INFECTION

Puerperal mastitis and lactating breast abscesses are now uncommon in developed countries but are still frequent problems in many parts of the world. The reasons for the decrease in frequency are improved maternal and infant hygiene, changes in breast-feeding patterns and earlier treatment of infection with appropriate antibiotics. *Staph. aureus* is usually the organism responsible although *Staph. epidermis* and streptococci are occasionally isolated.

Aetiology and pathogenesis

It remains uncertain whether the organisms responsible for lactating breast infection are derived from the skin of the patient herself or from the mouth of her suckling child. Infection is usually associated with a break in the skin, such as a cracked nipple. These skin breaks reduce local defence mechanisms and result in an increase in the number of bacteria in the area around the nipple. These bacteria then enter the breast through the nipple and not through breaks in the skin as has been previously suggested. When infection is present the involved portion of breast is often engorged with milk and drainage into major ducts is then poor. Whether problems with milk drainage result from blockage of a major breast duct or occur as a consequence of infection is unknown.

Clinical features

Infection associated with breast feeding is most common within the first month after delivery, although some women do develop infection associated with weaning. Presenting features include pain, swelling and tenderness (Fig. 4.1). In the later stages there may be a fluctuant mass with overlying shiny, red skin. Axillary lymphadenopathy is not usually a feature of lactating breast infection. Patients can be toxic with a pyrexia, tachycardia and leucocytosis.

Management

- Antibiotics administered early in puerperal mastitis can abort abscess formation. The antibiotics of choice are flucloxacillin (500 mg four times a day) or co-amoxyclav (375 mg three times a day). Tetracycline, ciprofloxacin and chloramphenicol should not be used as they enter breast milk and may do the child harm. Breast feeding should be continued as this promotes drainage of the engorged segment and helps resolve infection.
- As fluctuation can be a late sign of abscess formation, patients whose condition does not rapidly improve on antibiotic therapy should have needle aspiration performed over the point of maximum tenderness following application of a local anaesthetic (EMLA) cream which is left *in situ* for 1 h. If the overlying skin is normal this technique is both diagnostic and therapeutic. On average, between three and four aspirations are needed for most breast abscesses and this form of management produces an excellent final cosmetic outcome.

  If the overlying skin is thinned or necrotic, having drained the pus with a small incision, the cavity should be irrigated initially with local anaesthetic solution. This produces instant pain relief. Thereafter the cavity should be irrigated with saline.
- Few lactating abscesses require drainage under general anaesthesia and the placement of a drain after incision and drainage is not necessary. Patients who have incision and drainage of

their breast abscess under general anaesthesia usually have to stop breast feeding, but patients who are treated by mini-incision or aspiration and antibiotics can continue to breast feed if they wish. It is rarely necessary to suppress lactation in patients with breast infection.

NON-LACTATING INFECTION

These infections can be separated into those occurring centrally in the periareolar region and those affecting the peripheral breast tissue.

Periareolar infection

This predominantly affects young women with a mean age of 32 years and occurs in association with periductal mastitis. Histologically periductal mastitis is characterized by active inflammation around non-dilated ducts. There are often polymorphs and granulomas around an involved duct although the predominant cell is the plasma cell, which explains why one of the terms used for this condition has been plasma cell mastitis. The preferred terminology is periductal mastitis and this condition is separate from duct ectasia. Duct ectasia is associated with different clinical symptoms, has different pathological features and affects an older age group.

Aetiology and pathogenesis

Current evidence suggests that smoking is an important factor in the aetiology of this condition. Whether substances in cigarette smoke are concentrated in the ducts and these cause direct damage or whether the cigarette smoke causes vascular changes and causes damage to breast ducts is unclear. Smoking does however appear to induce damage to the subareolar ducts and there is frequently an area of necrotic duct which can then become infected. Bacteria including enterococci, anaerobic streptococci, *bacteroides species* and *Staph. aureus* have been isolated from lesions of periductal mastitis.

Clinical features

Patients may present initially with periareolar inflammation with or without a mass, an established abscess (Fig. 4.2) or a mammary duct fistula (Fig. 4.3).

PERIAREOLAR INFLAMMATION

Management

- Initial treatment is with appropriate antibiotics.
- If the mass fails to resolve, perform fine needle aspirate to exclude an underlying cancer and an ultrasound to determine if an abscess is present.
- If an abscess is present, treat as for a lactating abscess.

Infection associated with periductal mastitis is frequently recurrent and these episodes should be treated by excision of the diseased duct alone or a total duct excision, the operation being performed under antibiotic cover by an experienced breast surgeon.

PERIAREOLAR ABSCESS

- Treatment is for lactating breast abscesses with aspiration and antibiotics (co-amoxyclav) or mini-incision and drainage.
- Abscesses associated with periductal mastitis commonly recur because treatment by incision and drainage does not remove the underlying diseased duct.
- Up to one-third of patients following treatment for non-lactating abscess develop a mammary duct fistula.
- Recurrent episodes of infection require definitive duct surgery — either excision of the single diseased duct or a total duct excision.

MAMMARY DUCT FISTULA

Mammary duct fistula is a communication between the skin usually in the periareolar region and a major subareolar breast duct (Fig. 4.4).

Aetiology and pathogenesis

Periductal mastitis is the major cause of mammary duct fistula and may develop following incision and drainage of a non-lactating breast abscess; spontaneous discharge of a periareolar inflammatory mass; biopsy of an area of periductal mastitis, or incision and drainage of a non-lactating breast abscess.

Clinical features

There is a discharging fistula at the areolar margin usually associated with nipple retraction. The median age of patients with this

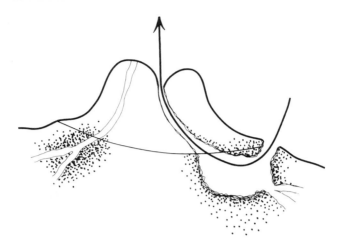

Fig. 4.4   A schematic diagram of a mammary duct fistula. At one side of the diagram a duct can be seen surrounded by numbers of black dots which represent periareolar inflammation. A biopsy of this area, incision and drainage if an abscess develops or spontaneous discharge, usually at the areolar margin, results in a mammary duct fistula seen on the other side of the diagram. Note the retracted nipple at the site of the involved duct.

problem is 35 years and over 90% are smokers. There have usually been preceding episodes of recurrent abscess formation and pussy discharge both through the nipple and through the fistula opening at the areolar margin. Occasionally there can be more than one opening at the areolar margin from a single involved duct.

Management

Treatment is surgical and consists of either opening up the fistula tract and leaving it to granulate, or excising the fistula and closing the wound primarily under antibiotic cover.

PERIPHERAL NON-LACTATING BREAST ABSCESSES

Aetiology and pathogenesis

Peripheral non-lactating breast abscesses are less common than periareolar abscesses, but they do occur and are often associated with an underlying disease state such as diabetes, rheumatoid arthritis, steroid treatment and trauma; they can also be associated with sebaceous cysts within the skin of the breast. Pilonidal abscesses in sheep shearers and barbers have also been reported. *Staph.*

aureus is the usual causative organism but some abscesses contain anaerobic organisms.

Clinical features

These abscesses are more common in premenopausal than post-menopausal women with a ratio of 3:1. Characteristically the patient presents with a lump which is tender and may be associated with inflammatory changes in the overlying skin of the breast. Systemic evidence of malaise or fever are usually absent. There may be a history of an underlying disease process and, if the abscess is secondary to a sebaceous cyst, a punctum may be identified.

Management

As for lactating periareolar abscesses with aspiration (Fig. 4.5) or incision and drainage.

SKIN ASSOCIATED INFECTION

Cellulitis of the skin of the breast with or without abscess formation is common, particularly in obese patients and/or those with large breasts. It also affects those who have poor breast hygiene. The lower half of the breast is most commonly affected, where the patient sweats and intertrigo develops. *Staph. aureus* and fungi are the most common organisms responsible for this infection. Skin infection can also be seen in association with sebaceous cysts and hidradenitis suppurativa.

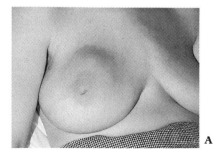

Fig. 4.5   Peripheral breast abscess before **(A)** and after **(B)** treatment by recurrent aspiration and oral antibiotics.

Treatment

- Weight reduction.
- Keep areas as clean and dry as possible — washing twice per day; avoid creams and talcum powder; use cotton bras or cotton T-shirt, or vest worn inside bra.
- Appropriate courses of antibiotics and antifungal powder.

OTHER RARE INFECTIONS

Tuberculosis

Tuberculosis is now rare and can be primary or secondary, but the latter is more common. In secondary tuberculosis, infection usually reaches the breast by lymphatic spread from axillary, mediastinal or cervical nodes, or from directly underlying structures such as rib and costochondral junction or pleura.

Clinical features

Tuberculosis predominantly affects women in the latter part of the childbearing period. As it is now rare in developed countries the diagnosis is difficult to make. A breast or axillary sinus is present in up to 50% of patients. The most common presentation is with an acute abscess which occurs as a result of infection of an area of tuberculosis by pyogenic organisms.

Management

- Establish diagnosis — may need biopsy.
- Combination of surgery and antituberculous drug therapy.

Syphilis, actinomycosis, mycotic, helminthic and viral infections occasionally affect the breast, but are rare.

Granulomatous lobular mastitis

This is probably a variant of periductal mastitis and is characterized by non-caseating granulomata and micro-abscesses confined to the breast.

Clinical features

Young parous women are most frequently affected. Organisms may be found in these lesions but do not appear to have a primary role in its aetiology.

Management

The diagnosis can often be established on fine needle aspiration cytology (FNAC) and surgery should be avoided if possible. When surgical intervention is performed, it is frequently followed by wound infection and, occasionally, a mammary duct fistula develops. There is a strong tendency for this condition to persist and recur. There is no specific treatment and the condition usually resolves spontaneously. The same antibiotics used in periductal mastitis have been tried without much success and corticosteroids have been advocated by some.

Factitial disease

Factitious abscesses may occasionaly be seen. These patients generally have psychiatric problems, but some can be quite plausible and the condition needs to be suspected where peripheral abscesses persist or recur after appropriate treatment. The condition may be difficult to treat as patients are often resistant to help and may be very manipulative.

DUCT ECTASIA

Definition and terminology

The conditions of periductal mastitis and duct ectasia, which are benign conditions affecting major breast ducts, are poorly understood and, unfortunately, the terms are often used interchangeably. It is now appreciated that there are almost certainly two separate conditions: periductal mastitis, which affects predominantly young women, and duct ectasia, which is probably an aberration of normal breast involution, affecting older women. It is the same condition that was first recognized in 1923 by Bloodgood when he referred to the variceal tumour of the breast because of the finding of palpable subareolar dilated ducts.

Incidence

Mammary duct ectasia is more common than is generally appreciated and in one autopsy series was found in 25% of normal female breasts. In the majority it does not produce any specific symptoms.

Clinical presentation

Patients can present with nipple discharge which may be from several ducts and is usually cheesy in nature or with a palpable mass which may be hard or doughy. Multiple duct, green-coloured discharge has often been said to be due to duct ectasia but this is physiological discharge and the underlying condition is not duct ectasia. Duct ectasia is the most common cause of nipple discharge in women over the age of 55 years.

Nipple retraction may be the sole presenting feature and may be associated with nipple discharge. Nipple retraction is classically slit-like with the central portion of the nipple being pulled in rather than the whole nipple. This separates it from nipple inversion, seen in association with severe inflammatory diseases where the whole nipple is pulled in. The mean age of patients with discharge is 53 years and retraction is bilateral in 15%. Of all benign masses, 3–4% are related to duct ectasia.

Pathology and aetiology

As a patient ages, the ducts dilate and shorten. Duct ectasia is no more than an aberration of this normal process. As the ducts dilate, they contain inspissated material but have minimal surrounding inflammation. Duct ectasia is not associated with previous episodes of inflammatory breast disease and is unrelated to smoking. Duct ectasia is a completely separate condition from periductal mastitis.

Management and treatment

- Patients with troublesome discharge should be treated surgically, usually by total duct excision.
- All patients with nipple inversion/retraction should be investigated with clinical examination and mammography.
- Patients with a clinical or mammographic suspicion require a cytological or histological diagnosis.

The majority of patients with duct ectasia require no specific treatment other than reassurance.

Breast cancer

5. Risk factors, screening and prevention

INTRODUCTION

Breast cancer is common, affecting one in 12 women and causing 21 000 deaths a year in the UK. The prevalence is around five times higher, and more than 70% of those with 'operable' disease will be alive and well 5 years after diagnosis.

The previous Government highlighted breast cancer as one of four 'key sites' in the cancer section of the recent plan of Health for the Nation. They intended to reduce the incidence of breast cancer detected through screening by 25% before the year 2000 (from 98 cases detected per 10 000 screened to 74). They encouraged those responsible for health care provision to extend the models of care developed for the screened population to the general, symptomatic patient. In addition, the Calman-Hine report on provision of cancer services stressed the need for surgical site specialization and an increase in non-surgical oncology with high quality services for the common cancers being provided close to the patient's residence.

Breast cancer is an emotive subject and there is a general fear that all lumps are malignant. This is not so — only one in eight breast lumps presenting to breast clinics are cancers.

Breast diseases, including cancer, are increasingly being treated in specialist units where close co-operation between interested surgeons, pathologists, radiologists and associated staff allow rapid and accurate diagnosis with appropriate treatment to be offered to patients. The trend for breast reconstruction and chemotherapy to be provided in the District General Hospital setting is also increasing with the patient needing to travel only for radiotherapy services. Specialist training for those interested in breast surgery is now underway and a specialist breast nurse (counsellor) has been appointed to all units dealing with breast diseases.

HISTORY

Breast cancer is not a new disease and was recorded by the Egyptians. Hippocrates and Celsus both describe some of the clinical features. Leonides was operating on malignant breast lumps at the end of the first century AD using cautery to both control bleeding and to eradicate remnants of the disease. Galen (c. 130 AD) exerted much influence on medical thought and laid down criteria for operative and conservative management; his ideas held sway until the 16th Century.

The patron saint of breast diseases is St Agatha, who was martyred having her breasts removed in Sicily, in the 3rd Century. There is extensive literature relating to breast cancer in the Middle Ages and the Renaissance with details of both conventional and some quite bizarre treatments (see **Further reading**).

RISK FACTORS FOR AND EPIDEMIOLOGY OF BREAST CANCER

Age

The risk of developing breast cancer increases with age. It is rare before the age of 25 but the incidence increases leading up to the menopause. There is a slight downward trend during the menopausal years (the menopausal hook of Clemmenson) before its incidence again continues to rise with advancing years although with a reduced rate (Fig. 5.1). Breast cancer accounts for almost 20% of all cancer deaths but, because of variations in the age distribution of different cancers, the proportion of deaths in different ages caused by breast cancer is highest between the ages of 44 and 50 following which it steadily declines (Fig. 5.2).

Geographic variation

There is a marked variation in the incidence of mortality of breast cancer between different countries (Fig. 5.3). Large increases in the rates of breast cancer occur in populations migrating from nations with a low incidence to those with a high incidence of breast cancer, indicating the existence of environmental factors.

Age at menarche and menopause

Women who start menstruating early in life or who have late menopause have an increased risk of developing breast cancer. Women who have a natural menopause after the age of 55 years have

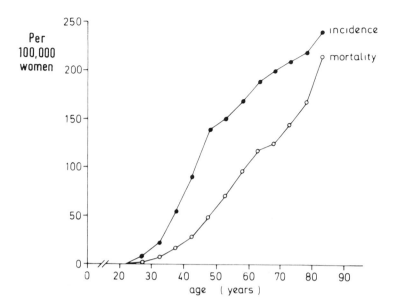

Fig. 5.1 Age-specific incidence and mortality of breast cancer.

twice the risk of developing breast cancer compared to women whose menopause occurs before the age of 45. In the extreme, women who undergo a bilateral oophorectomy before the age of 35 have a 40% higher risk of breast cancer than those who have a natural menopause (Table 5.1).

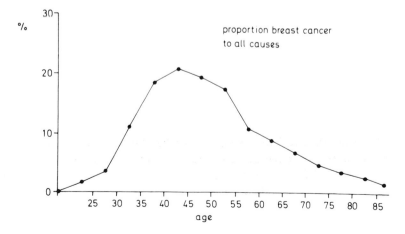

Fig. 5.2 Percentage of all deaths at different ages due to breast cancer.

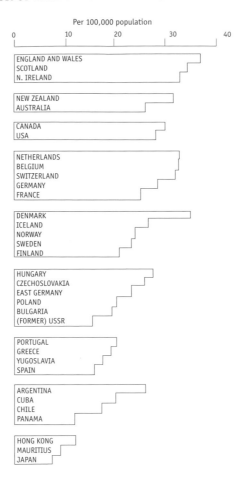

Fig. 5.3   Female breast cancer mortality incidence in different parts of the world.

Age at first pregnancy

Nulliparity and late age at first birth both increase the lifetime incidence of breast cancer. The risk of breast cancer in women who have their first child after the age of 30 is about twice that of women who have their first child before the age of 20. Women who have their first child after the age of 35 appear to be at even higher risk than nulliparous women (Table 5.1). An earlier age at the birth of a second child further reduces the risk of breast cancer.

Table 5.1   Established and probable risk factors for breast cancer

Risk factor	Comparison category	Risk category	Typical relative risk
Age at menarche	16 years	11–14 years	1.3
		15 years	1.1
Age at menopause	45–54 years	After 55 years	1.5
		Before 45 years	0.7
		Oophorectomy before 35 years	0.4
Age at birth of first child	Before 20 years	20–24 years	1.3
		25–29 years	1.6
		30 years	1.9
		Nulliparous	1.9
Family history of breast cancer	No first-degree relatives affected	Mother affected before age of 60	2.0
		Mother affected after age of 60	1.4
		Two first-degree relatives affected	4.0–6.0
Benign breast disease	No evidence of proliferation change	Proliferation only	2.0
		Atypical hyperplasia	4.5
Alcohol use	Non-drinker	1 drink/day	1.4
		2 drinks/day	1.7
		3 drinks/day	2.0
Radiation	No special exposure	Atomic bomb (100 rad)	3.0
		Repeated fluoroscopy	1.5–2.0
Oral contraceptive use	Never used	Current use*	1.5
		Prolonged use before first pregnancy	2.0
		Past use	1.0
Postmenopausal oestrogen replacement therapy	Never used	<5 years use	1.04
		10 years use	1.13
		15 years use	1.27

*Relative risks may be higher for women with a diagnosis of breast cancer before the age of 40

Lactation

Initial studies suggested that breast feeding for at least 3 months reduced the risk of breast cancer by 22% per baby fed, but more recent and larger studies have indicated that breast feeding may not provide a significant degree of protection against breast cancer.

Family history

Up to 10% of breast cancer in Western countries is due to genetic predisposition. Breast cancer susceptibility is generally inherited as an autosomal dominance with limited penetrance. This means that it can be transmitted through either sex and some family members may transmit the abnormal gene without developing breast cancer themselves. It is not yet known how many breast cancer genes there are, about one-third of familial cases are thought to be due to mutation in the first breast cancer gene discovered, BRCA1, which is on the long arm of chromosome 17. This is a large gene with over 200 described mutations which are widely spread across the gene. Some BRCA1 mutations may be associated with different risks of breast cancer. Mutations early in the gene predispose to ovarian and breast cancer whereas mutations in the distal portion of the gene are associated almost exclusively with breast cancer. There are some specific mutations that occur with specific groups such as the deletion of the A-G at position 185 found in Aschkenazy Jews. The second hereditary breast cancer locus, BRCA2, has been identified on the long arm of chromosome 13. This seems to be associated with families which contain males with breast cancer. In addition, a few cases arise from mutations in p53 gene on the short arm of chromosome 17. There is also evidence that the ataxia telangectasia gene may also be important in relation to breast cancer. Of particular concern is that patients with this gene may be more sensitive to radiation and that repeated mammography may induce some cancers.

Some families affected by breast cancer show an excess of other cancers including ovary and prostate. Women most likely to be carrying an inherited gene are those who develop breast cancer at an early age or those who develop a combination of breast cancer and another epithelial cancer. Most breast cancers that are due to a genetic mutation occur before the age of 65 and a women with a strong family history of breast cancer of early onset who does not develop the disease by the age of 65 has probably not inherited the genetic mutation.

A woman's risk of breast cancer is two or more times greater if she has a first-degree relative (mother, sister or daughter) who develops breast cancer before the age of 50 and the younger the relative at the time she developed breast cancer, the greater the risk. For example, a women whose sister developed breast cancer at age 39 has a cumulative risk of 10–15% of developing the disease herself by the age of 65, but that risk is only 5% (only just above the population risk) if her sister was aged 50–54 at diagnosis. Risk increases by four to six times if two first-degree relatives develop the disease. For example, a woman with two affected relatives, one of whom was aged 50 at diagnosis has a 25% chance of developing breast cancer by the age of 65.

Relative risk for invasive breast cancer in patients with benign disease

Women with palpable breast cysts, duct papillomas, sclerosing adenosis, moderate florid epithelial hyperplasia and previous benign disease do have some increased risk of breast cancer compared to those without these changes. The risk is, however, not of the order that is clinically significant. The relative risk for invasive cancer in patients with benign disease is shown in Table 5.2.

Weight

Obesity is not a major risk factor for breast cancer. Among premenopausal women it is actually associated with a reduced incidence of breast cancer. However, in postmenopausal women body mass index greater than 35 is associated with up to two times relative risk of developing breast cancer. This is because fat is an important source of oestrogen production in postmenopausal women and obese women have higher oestrogen levels.

Diet

Evidence implicating diet in the aetiology of breast cancer includes the observation that fat may cause mammary tumours in rodents,

Table 5.2 Relative risk for invasive breast cancer in patients with benign disease

Risk	Disease type
No increased risk	Mild hyperplasia Duct ectasia Apocrine metaplasia Simple fibroadenoma Microcysts Periductal mastitis Adenosis
Slight increased risk 1.5–2 times	Gross cysts Moderate and florid hyperplasia Papilloma Sclerosing adenosis Complex fibroadenoma
Moderately increased risk 4–5 times	Atypical hyperplasia

and that mortality from breast cancer in different countries strongly correlates with the corresponding per capita fat consumption. Studies of total fat have, however, not found that women with breast cancer report a significantly higher consumption than controls, and the relationship may simply reflect total calorific intake rather than just fat intake. No definitive conclusion can therefore be drawn from the data currently available. Some studies have suggested that green vegetables may have a protective effect against breast cancer but this requires confirmation.

Alcohol intake

Alcohol consumption, even at the level of one drink per day, has been associated with a moderate increased risk of breast cancer in the majority of studies (Table 5.1).

Radiation

Exposure to ionizing radiation, particularly between puberty and the age of 30, can substantially increase the risk of breast cancer. However, exposure to clinically important levels is rare.

Oral contraceptive pill

A recent meta-analysis of all the published studies of oral contraceptives and breast cancer risk has shown that there is a relative risk of developing breast cancer of 1.3 while patients are taking the oral contraceptive pill and this risk persists for up to 10 years after stopping the pill. The cancers which develop in women on the pill are, however, more likely to be localized to the breast and less likely to involve regional nodes. Considering the benefits of the pill this slight increased risk is not considered clinically significant and may be due to the fact that women who are on the oral contraceptive pill are more likely to be examined at regular intervals and so breast cancer is more likely to be detected.

Postmenopausal oestrogen replacement therapy

Use of hormone replacement therapy (HRT) appears to increase the risk of breast cancer for individuals taking it, but this risk disappears within 5 years of stopping these preparations. The risk of developing breast cancer is offset by the benefits of prophylaxis against osteoporosis and ischaemic heart disease (although the benefit for the latter has recently been questioned). Current cost-benefit analysis indicates that up to 10 years' HRT has significant advantages. Data on more prolonged use are scanty, but do suggest that there may be a significant risk of breast cancer in women who are on hormone replacement beyond 15 years (Table 5.3). Combining progesterone with oestrogen replacement reduces the risk of endometrial cancer but does not appear to decrease the risk of breast cancer and may even add to it.

There is no evidence that HRT has a greater effect on women who are otherwise at increased risk of breast cancer. HRT in these women may therefore be appropriate if the woman is experiencing significant menopausal symptoms. There are other agents which have been shown to be effective for menopausal symptoms, particularly progestogens (megestrol acetate 20 mg twice a day) which are effective at treating hot flushes and local oestrogen preparations such as Vagifem for vaginal dryness.

Cigarette smoking

Current evidence suggests there may be a small negative link between breast cancer incidence and smoking but any effect is very small.

SCREENING

Introduction

Screening is the presumptive identification of unrecognized disease by the application of tests, examinations or other procedures which can be applied rapidly. Presumptive is the important word because all screening does is identify two groups of individuals, test positive and test negative. Those who are test positive require a series of diagnostic investigations to determine whether they do truly have the disease being sought, whereas those who are test negative should not need to be further investigated.

Table 5.3 Additional breast cancer cases that might be expected for different durations of HRT started at age 50. Background risk at this age is 40 cases per 100 population

Duration of HRT	Additional cases per 1000
5 years	2
10 years	6
15 years	12

Screening tests should:

- Be simple to apply.
- Be cheap.
- Be easy to perform.
- Be easy and unambiguous to interpret.
- Have the ability to define those with disease.
- Exclude those without disease.

Mammography:

- Is expensive.
- Requires high technology and machinery.
- Requires special film and processing.
- Requires highly trained radiologists to interpret the films.
- Detects only 95% of all breast cancers at best and only half those lesions detected are malignant.

Mammography is, however, the best screening tool available for the detection of breast cancer and, in fact, is the only screening modality for any malignancy for which the value has been demonstrated by rigorous randomized trials.

Evidence that screening is effective

A number of randomized trials have been undertaken in Europe and the USA and, in addition, there have been a number of non-randomized, population-based screening programmes (such as in the UK). There is considerable agreement among trials in showing a reduction in breast cancer mortality between the ages of 50 and 70 (Fig. 5.4). For women over the age of 50 trials indicate an average reduction in mortality of 29%. If one actually estimates the reduction in mortality in those who attend screening then it is estimated that 40% of breast cancer deaths in the attenders can be delayed or prevented. This translates into a 1–2% reduction in overall mortality for women over the age of 50 years.

Compliance, that is the percentage of those invited for screening who attend, is a major factor influencing the effectiveness of screening and, as compliance falls, so do the benefits of screening.

Characteristics of screen-detected cancers

When compared with patients presenting with symptomatic breast cancers, breast carcinomas detected by screening are more likely to be small, *in situ* rather than invasive and the invasive cancers are

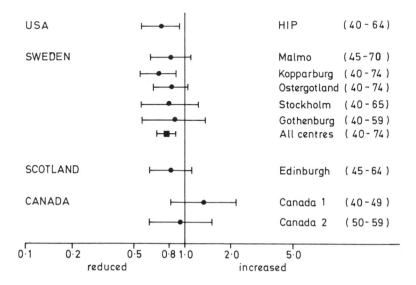

Fig. 5.4   Summary of 7–12-year mortality data in randomized trials of breast cancer screening. The dots represent the absolute reduction in mortality found within each study and the lines emanating from each dot represent the confidence limits. Where the confidence limits do not cross 0, then the reduction in mortality is significant. HIP = Health Insurance Plan.

more likely to be better differentiated and of 'special type'. Screen-detected cancers are also more likely to be node negative than symptomatic cancers of the same size (Fig. 5.5). The ability of screening to detect cancers at a very early stage and to influence subsequent mortality indicates that early diagnosis and appropriate treatment of breast cancer reduces the chance of metastatic disease being present.

Overdiagnosis of breast cancer

Some well-differentiated invasive cancers and a number of *in situ* cancers would almost certainly not have caused symptoms during the patient's lifetime. There are no indications from the currently available data that invasive breast carcinomas are being overdiagnosed by screening. It is possible that a number of cases of *in situ* carcinoma are detected by screening which would not become clinically significant and this perhaps results in unnecessary treatment in these individuals. Until more is known of the natural history of carcinoma *in situ*, the extent to which this diagnosis and subsequent over-treatment actually occurs during a screening programme remains unknown.

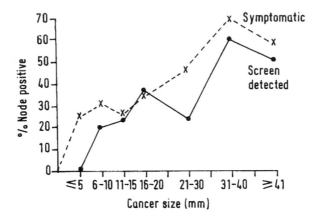

Fig. 5.5 Relationship of node positivity rate to tumour size for screen-detected and symptomatic breast cancers.

Recommendations for screening

Age range

Current available data indicate that the reduction in mortality is maximal between the age of 50 and 70 years. There is no evidence to support screening in younger women because the incidence of breast cancer is less frequent in younger women and mammography has a decreased sensitivity, detecting only two-thirds of breast cancers present in women under the age of 50.

Frequency of screening

The most appropriate interval between mammographic screens has yet to be determined. Although from a cost-benefit point of view (cost per year of life gained and cost of quality-adjusted year of life saved) 3-yearly screening of women aged 50–64 years of age appears to be the most cost-effective screening policy, the interval cancer rate climbs rapidly between the second and third year after the initial screen, suggesting that this 3-year interval is too long. In contrast, annual screening is almost certainly too frequent and the optimum frequency for screening is probably 2 years.

Number of mammographic views

Studies have suggested that all patients should have two views at the first screen but only one view subsequently. This is now standard practice for the NHS Breast Screening Programme. Some units are performing two views (oblique and craniocaudal) even for interval screens.

Methods of screening

There is no evidence that screening using clinical examination, breast ultrasound or the teaching of breast self examination are effective tools for screening for breast cancer.

Breast self examination. There is evidence that women who perform regular breast self examination detect smaller tumours than those who do not. The problem with breast self examination is that it needs to be taught by experienced personnel and this is costly. Furthermore, only 30–50% of women who are invited to be taught breast self examination attend and little is known of the extent to which women comply and continue to practise breast self examination. Of those studies which have evaluated breast self examination as a screening tool, none has shown a significant reduction in mortality in those women invited to be taught breast self examination. There are also concerns that regular breast self examination induces anxiety amongst women who practise it and results in an increase in the number of benign breast masses detected which then subsequently require assessment.

While women should be encouraged to examine their own breasts and get to know their 'lumps and bumps', it is clear that it is not worthwhile investing money in teaching women regular breast self examination.

Screening of high-risk groups

Although there is no evidence that regular screening of patients at high risk of breast cancer who are outwith the age range of 50–70 years actually benefits in terms of overall reduction in mortality, a number of units throughout the country offer specific groups regular breast screening.

Family history

For patients who are either at a relative risk of greater than 2.5 times that of the general population, many units are now offering regular mammographic screening for women on an annual basis starting 5–10 years younger than the age at which the youngest relative has developed breast cancer. Although there is no national funding, some units are offering patients who are considered on the basis of their family history to be at very high risk, genetic screening and testing for the BRCA1 gene under very strict conditions.

HRT

The consensus view is that women do not require mammography prior to starting HRT although all women should have a full clinical examination before HRT is instituted. Most women on HRT should not be screened more regularly or at an earlier age than is currently available within the Government screening programme. For women who start HRT below the age of 40 and are on it for longer than 10 years, the current recommendations are that these women should start being screened after 10 years on HRT by mammography, performed at 2-yearly intervals. HRT may increase the breast density and lower the sensitivity of mammography (Fig 2.10, p. 16).

Patients with atypical hyperplasia

Current recommendations are that these women should be screened every 1–2 years as for women with a family history, 2-yearly from age 35–40 and annually from age 40–50. After the age of 50, screening at 18-monthly intervals is probably most appropriate.

Gene testing

To test an individual it must first be possible to demonstrate that there is an abnormal gene in the family. The family history indicates the likely presence of an inherited gene. The search usually begins with an affected relative who has developed breast cancer and one of the two breast cancer genes, BRCA1 or BRCA2, are screened for common mutations. If an abnormal gene is found then the same abnormality should be sought in another family member before the test is offered to an unaffected relative. This allows confirmation that the mutation is not sporadic in nature. Only then is it possible to gene test other members of the family. Before genetic testing any individual needs to be seen and counselled on at least two separate occasions and the individual made aware of the implications not only for her but her immediate relatives of both a positive and a negative test. Options if the test is positive also need to be discussed. If the individual then opts for gene testing, blood is removed and a date arranged for the person to return for the result. The test result is given directly to the individual and a post-test, follow-up appointment arranged. Both positive and negative tests are associated with significant problems. A person who has a negative test often feels guilty that they have not been affected. There are major implications with regard to life insurance and taking out a mortgage for patients who test gene positive.

The options for individuals shown to carry the gene are regular screening, bilateral prophylactic mastectomy and entering one of the ongoing prevention trials.

Initial figures suggested that carriers of a gene such as BRCA1 had an 80–85% chance of developing breast cancer, but more recent studies have suggested that the risk of developing breast cancer in carriers is considerably less and may be of the order of 50%.

Bilateral subcutaneous mastectomy — prophylactic

This operation was devised to allow the breast tissue to be resected whilst sparing the skin and nipple, thus allowing a reconstruction to be offered. Before genetic testing was available some patients requested the operation on the basis of family history alone. There has been reluctance to perform this surgery as the cosmetic results were not always satisfactory and there were concerns about the amount of breast tissue that might be left behind. A subcutaneous mastectomy may leave appreciable amounts of breast tissue which potentially remains at 100% of the risk of developing cancer. Improved techniques and appropriate incisions with concentration of this type of surgery in the hands of experts has increased its acceptability. Alternatives for reconstruction include placement of prostheses or de-epithelized flaps.

Some patients also have prophylactic oophorectomy.

Summary of criteria for referral to family history clinic

- All screening and treatment of individuals at high risk should be part of a clinically audited programme.
- Mammography (initial two view then single oblique) should start at the age of 35 years, or 5 years younger than the youngest affected family member (whichever is youngest), biannual mammography up to the age of 40 and annual clinical examination.
- Between the ages of 40–50 years these women should have annual mammography and clinical examination.
- At ages greater than 50 years dependent on risk either: discharge to NHSBSP; or contact 18 monthly (high risk families only).

A trial of magnetic resonance imaging (MRI) of patients at risk because of family history is underway.

PREVENTION OF BREAST CANCER

The idea that the incidence of breast cancer might be reduced by intervention is not new. Hormonal manipulation by means of oophorectomy was proposed in the 1930s but did not gain favour! More recently the observation that, during trials of tamoxifen as adjuvant treatment for breast cancer, the observed number of second breast cancers was less than expected, indicated that this agent might be used to reduce breast cancer incidence. A study to compare tamoxifen with placebo taken for 5 years in women (not patients) with risk factors for development of breast cancer (IBIS) is underway in the UK and other countries.

Other measures that have been proposed to reduce the incidence of breast cancer include reduction of dietary fat intake. This would be difficult to achieve without major socio-cultural changes and would probably be opposed by some groups of food producers.

The retinoids are an interesting group of compounds which have effects on the growth and differentiation of epithelial cells. There is both *in vivo* and *in vitro* experimental work which suggests that they may have a role in cancer prevention, and a clinical trial of one of the retinoid family is underway.

Other possible preventative agents include selenium, which has not yet been subject to controlled trials.

When considering trials of cancer prevention one has to take account of the number of subjects needed to demonstrate an effect and the type of prevention being planned. Individuals have different risks depending on the extent of their family history of breast cancer and the nature of any previous breast disease. Thus to detect a reduction in relative risk from 3.0 (as might be expected in those at risk with a strong family history) to 2.5, a sample size of approximately 100 000 would be needed; whereas if the intervention reduced the risk to 1.5 then the sample would only need to be around 9500.

A report from Guy's Hospital has suggested that there might be a benefit from operating on patients with breast cancer in the second half of their menstrual cycle. During the first half of the cycle there is a phase of unopposed oestrogen and experimental work with mice has shown that operating during this phase leads to diminished survival. This retrospective study has been repeated in various centres with conflicting results. Many find no effect at all and some others find a significant result in the opposite direction. Since the size of the effect is potentially so great that it would outweigh the benefits of chemotherapy, a prospective study has been set up and is currently recruiting patients.

6. Pathology, prognosis, diagnosis and treatment

PATHOLOGY OF BREAST CANCER

Breast cancer arises in the terminal duct lobular unit. Breast cancer was originally described according to its macroscopic appearances and words like scirrhous (meaning woody) still unfortunately appear in the literature. More recently, breast cancer has been classified according to histological features; the modern classification is shown in Table 6.1. The division into invasive ductal and invasive lobular types is unfortunate as it is clear that cancers arise in the terminal duct lobular unit (rather than ductal carcinomas arising in the ducts and lobular carcinomas in the lobules). As the terms 'invas-

Table 6.1 Histological classification of breast cancer and frequency of presentation in a symptomatic population

History	% frequency
Non-invasive	
Ductal carcinoma *in situ*	6
Lobular carcinoma *in situ*	0.2
Invasive	
No special type, 'ductal carcinoma'	68
Special types	
Lobular	
classical	3
variants	7
Tubular	3
Cribriform	3
Medullary	3
Mucinous	2
Microinvasive	2
Papillary	1
Other rare types*	1.8

*includes a few pure apocrine cancers, metaplastic cancers and adenoidcystic cancers

ive ductal' and 'lobular' are in common usage we continue to refer to them. A more logical classification is into special and no special type (NST) as different prognoses are seen. Many of the special types have a better prognosis.

Invasive carcinoma of NST — frequently called invasive ductal carcinoma — is the most common type accounting for up to 85% of all breast cancers. Special types include invasive lobular carcinoma (classical and variants), invasive tubular, cribriform, medullary and mucinous, with other types being uncommon.

Carcinoma cells confined to within the terminal duct lobular unit and the adjacent ducts, but which have not yet invaded through the basement membrane, are known as carcinoma *in situ*. As with invasive disease, two main types have been described — ductal carcinoma *in situ* (DCIS) and lobular carcinoma *in situ* (LCIS) (Table 6.1). Certain types of DCIS are associated with characteristic microcalcifications giving rise to a typical mammographic pattern. Comedo DCIS is the type of DCIS most likely to be associated with microcalcifications and is often localized, whilst the cribriform and micropapillary type tends to be multifocal. Some authors prefer to classify DCIS as large cell or small cell type (in a similar manner to lung cancer). Whereas LCIS tends to occur in pure form, DCIS often occurs as a mixture of the different types — comedo, cribriform, (micro)papillary and solid.

Invasive ductal carcinomas surrounded by an extensive intraduct component (EIC) are more likely to be multifocal and to need much wider excision in order to achieve clear resection margins. Patients who have a combination of involved margins and an extensive *in situ* component have an unacceptable rate of local recurrence following breast-conservation surgery.

The breast may be the site of secondaries from other malignancies (such as a lymphoma); these patients require different assessment and treatment and will not be discussed further.

For further details of these histological subtypes and their characteristic features a specialist textbook on breast pathology should be consulted (see **Further reading**).

Many more patients with DCIS are now being diagnosed during breast screening. Prior to the institution of breast screening, DCIS was uncommon and accounted for 5% or less of malignancies. However, with the advent of screening, there has been a surprising increase in frequency particularly over the past decade. In 1983 there was an estimated 4900 cases of DCIS in the USA but a decade later the number had increased to 23 368. This increase has been across all age groups with a 12% annual increase in the 30–39 year age group and a 15% annual increase in women over the age of 50. Is this increase in DCIS real and, if so, will it result in the reduction of the subsequent incidence of invasive cancer? Does it represent overdiagnosis of previously unrecognized atypical hyperplastic lesions?

Studies of diagnostic consistency have indicated that it is at the interface of DCIS and atypical hyperplasia that there is most variation between individual pathologists. A lesion measuring <3 mm in size is more likely to be atypical ductal hyperplasia (ADH) than DCIS and should be diagnosed as such. Some ADH lesions are larger, but those over 6 mm are rarely examples of ADH. Diagnostic consistency is much greater in large and high/intermediate grade DCIS which constitute the majority of such cases. So only a small percentage of the increase in incidence of DCIS seen over the last decade in the USA is likely to represent overdiagnosis. Whether the increase and detection of these early lesions will reduce the subsequent incidence of invasive cancer is not yet evident, although it is likely to do so.

Invasive ductal carcinomas surrounded by an extensive *in situ* component are often more difficult to remove and great care needs to be taken to ensure that both the cancer and the extensive *in situ* component are excised and clear resection margins are obtained.

Handling of the specimen

The pathologist should receive the specimen as soon as possible after surgery — in centres where research is undertaken fresh tissue is taken for study. Routine specimens are fixed in a formalin-containing solution prior to trimming and embedding in paraffin wax. These blocks are then cut with a microtome and stained to allow cellular detail to be examined (Fig. 6.1). Sections should be taken of the main specimen, resection margins and 'normal' non-involved tissue. The edges of a lumpectomy specimen may be painted with Indian ink to allow the involvement of resection margins to be assessed.

If the specimen is a mastectomy then sections of skin and nipple are also examined. If an axillary dissection is included then the nodes need to be carefully removed and examined individually. This takes time and skill but is important as decisions on adjuvant treatment are based on the result. The number of nodes reported to have been retrieved is often more a function of the pathologist's skill than the surgeon!

Routine reporting

The pathologist is in the best position to give the size of the lesion — clinical estimation is inaccurate although ultrasound can be used to reduce error. Size is an important prognostic factor and, coupled with nodal status and grade, can be used to form a prognostic index.

The tumour is assessed for grade using a technique known as Bloom and Richardson grading, named after the first two authors who described it. It is referred to as Scarff-Bloom grading in Europe and has been modified since its original description. Its use was initially resisted as inter-observer variation was high but it has now been standardized and is very reproducible. The grades are I–III and are made up of three components which are each numerically scored out of three. These are tubular differentiation, nuclear pleomorphism and the number of mitotic figures present. The higher the score the less well differentiated the tumour. The scores are summated to give a possible range of 3–9. Tumours with a score of 3, 4 or 5 are grade I; 6 and 7 grade II, and those scoring 8 and 9 are grade III. Grade alone is an important independent indicator of survival with 85% of patients with a grade I tumour being alive and well at 5 years compared to only a 45% 5-year survival in patients with a grade III lesion. This grading system is designed for use with carcinomas of NST (ductal carcinomas) and should not be used for lobular lesions which are described as low or high grade.

Vascular and lymphatic invasion by tumour can be assessed and is a poor prognostic sign if present. The presence of a round-cell infiltrate into the tumour edge is also assessed but gives less useful information as does the degree of elastosis.

The presence of EIC in an invasive cancer (defined as present if >25% of the main tumour mass is DCIS and if DCIS is present elsewhere in the surrounding tissue) is sought. Many would regard a report of EIC in the original excision specimen as an indication for further excision or a mastectomy if there was a report of EIC in the original biopsy or wide local excision specimen.

Nodal status is of paramount importance and is the gold standard against which other prognostic factors are compared and by which newer factors are judged. A discussion of the clinical importance of nodal status is given in the section on treatment of breast cancer. The pathologist not only has to dissect out the nodes but also examine them carefully. Tumour may only be present in small areas such as the subcapsular space, and it takes time to find these areas.

Attempts to improve this process by using a panel of monoclonal antibodies to stain these microdeposits have been tried. They reduce the time that the pathologist needs to spend at the microscope but at the expense of extra preparation and technician time. These techniques do allow more accurate definition of nodal status and identify some patients who would have been classified as node negative as, in fact, being node positive.

Special tests

Specialist tests such as oestrogen receptor, progesterone receptor and other putative histochemical markers of prognosis may be assayed. These are increasingly been performed by immunohistochemical techniques using specific monoclonal antibodies raised against the epitope of interest. Examples of these tests are:

- Oestrogen receptor.
- Progesterone receptor.
- Epidermal growth factor receptor.
- Ki-67.
- erb-B2.
- Cathepsin D.
- nm23.

Although most of them are of research interest, their introduction may allow identification of subgroups of patients who either require no adjuvant treatment or need a more aggressive approach.

Some breast neoplasms do not fall into the clear diagnostic groups considered earlier and special tests to determine their nature may be needed. These include special histological stains and the use of monoclonal antibodies.

PROGNOSTIC FACTORS

Survival of patients with breast cancer depends on two different groups of factors: tumour stage, reflecting chronology (i.e. how long the tumour has been present) and biological factors representing the biology or aggressiveness of the tumour.

The search for differential characteristics that allow one to determine a patient's outcome has been the subject of much research. As 50% of women with early breast cancer will be cured by surgery alone, or in combination with radiotherapy, there is a need to define these patients in order to spare them further therapy. Many factors have been proposed but few have stood the test of time or rigorous analysis. What works for one set of patients often fails to transfer to a different cohort. The criteria for a prognostic factor to be clinically accepted is outlined below.

The factor must:

- Have biological relevance.
- Be reproducible in different laboratories.
- Be validated prospectively in a large series of patients.
- Be confirmed independently by other workers.

In addition, they must have an appropriate cut-off point; must identify a population at high (or low) risk (there also needs to be an appropriate therapy which this population can be offered), and, ideally, they should be cheap and give an answer quickly. Many candidates have been proposed for prognostic factors and these are listed under **Special tests** (see page 107).

Prognostic factors may be divided into those obtained routinely (such as size, grade, nodal status) and those needing special biochemical or immunohistochemical tests.

Nodal status

The single 'gold standard' against which all other factors should be compared is nodal status. The more nodes involved the worse the prognosis (Fig. 6.2) with an average 10-year survival of 60–70% for node-negative patients dropping to 20–30% for those with involved nodes; adjuvant chemotherapy is now routinely given to premenopausal women in this group. There are probably subgroups of high-risk, node-negative patients who would also benefit from adjuvant chemotherapy.

Histology

Overall tumours of certain special type (classical lobular, tubular, cribriform, medullary, mucinous and papillary) have a much better prognosis than tumours of NST. This association appears independent of grade. Invasive carcinoma of tubular and cribriform types are associated with an excellent long-term survival and few patients with these tumours die as a result of their disease. Invasive medullary carcinomas are unusual tumours in that, according to the Bloom and Richardson classification, they are grade III and yet they are associated with a very much better prognosis than grade III NST carcinomas. In a series of patients from Edinburgh, the 5-year survival for patients with tumours of these

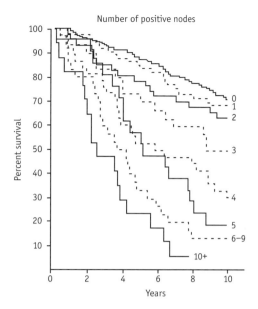

Fig. 6.2   Patients survival in relation to the
number of axillary nodes involved.

special types was 91% compared with 47% for carcinomas of NST.
Of patients alive 20 years after treatment for breast cancer, over
40% of long-term survivors had tumours of these special types
which is more than twice the percentage (15%) of all breast cancers
which are of these types.

Size

Size is a crude predictor of the metastatic potential of a tumour —
larger tumours having a higher incidence of metastasis to the
regional nodes. Even small tumours may have nodal involvement
(about 17% of those tumours smaller than 1 cm are node positive)
but generally most women with tumours measuring less than 1 cm
and negative nodes have an excellent prognosis.

Tumour grade

Tumour grade as assessed by the Bloom and Richardson system has
the ability to predict outcome with 86% of patients with grade I
tumours being alive at 5 years compared to 57% of those with a
grade III lesion.

These three factors may be combined to form a prognostic index which allows greater separation of survival curves. The best known of these indices is that defined by the Nottingham group based on a retrospective multivariate analysis of many hundred cases where survival and time to relapse was well quantified (Nottingham Prognostic Index [NPI]). They combined tumour grade, nodal status and size in the formula:

NPI = (0.2 x size cm) + grade + stage

to give a figure. Grade was assessed by the Bloom and Richardson method and scored 1–3. Stage was based on nodal status and was the combination of a triple-node biopsy (the low axilla, high axilla and internal mammary chain). They have shown this index works in a second, prospectively collected cohort and use it routinely to determine which patients need no further treatment after excision and radiotherapy. This index has been shown to be reproducible and even to work in Yorkshire! (Fig. 6.3). In Nottingham the tumours were all graded by one pathologist whereas in Yorkshire they were graded by a number of pathologists suggesting that grading is not as difficult as was once suggested. The Yorkshire surgeons adopted a more pragmatic approach to assessing nodes and did not (like most centres) perform internal mammary sampling.

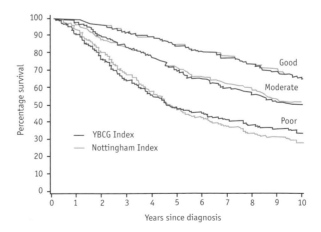

Fig. 6.3 Comparison of the Nottingham and Yorkshire Breast Cancer Group prognostic indices. Nottingham (NPI) score: good = <3.4; moderate = 3.4–5.4; poor = >5.4. Yorkshire (YBCG) score: good = <1.21; moderate = 1.2–1.82; poor = >1.82.

Newer biological factors

Other factors related to the biology of the tumour have been described. There are problems with standardization and inter-laboratory variation for many. Quality Assurance schemes have been implemented for some of the more important ones under the auspices of groups such as the European Organization for Research and Treatment of Cancer (EORTC). In the USA, where much more attention is paid to these factors, commercial assay of multiple factors has become big business. Many are still experimental and further work is needed before their place is established; many are not routinely measured in the UK as treatment decisions are made on the basis of more conventional factors.

Oestrogen receptor (ER)

ER status was the first of the 'biological' markers to be studied. Approximately 60% of tumours contain detectable ER. The original assay methods were biochemical using a radioligand assay but have now been replaced with immunocytochemical assays using a monoclonal antibody raised against an ER-related protein. Its initial promise as a useful discriminent has not held up — there is only a 5–10% difference in disease-free survival between patients with node-negative, ER-positive tumours and those with node-negative, ER-negative tumours. The survival after first relapse is, however, predicted by ER status with ER-positive patients living longer and having a better response to therapy be it chemotherapy or endocrine treatment. It is now recommended that all patients have their ER status estimated and recorded.

Progesterone receptor (PR)

PRs have been described and depend upon an intact ER pathway in order to be expressed. Their presence therefore tends to correlate with ER status but does allow definition of a subgroup of ER-positive patients with a better prognosis.

Cell kinetics and ploidy

Ploidy is a measurement of the relative proportion of DNA in each cell and can be combined with measurements of the rate of cell growth and division. The percentage of cells in active cell division (S-phase) can be determined by flow cytometry. S-phase is a better predictor of relapse and survival than ploidy but both can be used to good effect in the node-negative woman. Diploid tumours have a lower risk of relapse than aneuploid ones and low S-phase tumours have a more favourable prognosis regardless of ploidy. These analyses can be performed in both fresh and paraffin-embedded tissue. The use of the antibody Ki-67 allows an easier estimation of proliferation.

erb-B2

This protein is a cell membrane receptor and is the product of the *neu* oncogene. It has a similarity to epidermal growth factor receptor and can be detected in both paraffin-embedded and frozen sections by immunohistochemistry. There are problems in deciding whether a tumour should be classified as positive or negative. Node-positive women (already candidates for adjuvant therapy) with increased expression of erb-B2 fare less well; but the situation is less clear for those with node-negative tumours. erb-B2 has been used in conjunction with other prognostic factors and generally in each subset those with erb-B2-positive tumours have a worse outcome. There is a suggestion that patients with erb-B2-positive tumours may respond better to an anthracycline-containing chemotherapy regimen. Antibodies to the erb-B2 receptor are in clinical trials.

Epidermal growth factor receptor (EGFr)

This is another cell membrane protein which is related to an onco-gene product (v-erb-B — originally named after the erythroblastic virus which caused cancer in chickens). Binding of its ligand (EGF) promotes growth of cancer cells including breast cancer cells grown in culture. The presence of EGFrs correlates with other prognostic factors and there is a relationship between its presence and high grade (Bloom and Richardson grade III), and other indicators of poor outlook. EGFr does not correlate with nodal status and can be used to divide node-negative patients into two groups with good separation of survival curves. It has been added to the Nottingham Prognostic Index to increase its power. It has also been correlated directly with survival and is a predictor of a reduced disease-free and overall survival. EGFr also correlates with response to endocrine therapy — elderly patients treated with tamoxifen alone were five times more likely to respond if their tumours were EGFr negative.

Cathepsin D

This is one member of a family of proteases whose activity is stimulated by oestrogens. It may contribute to metastasis by dissolving basement membrane and extracellular matrix thus allowing cancer cells to spread. There is a good correlation between presence of cathepsin D and prognosis, with some studies showing that patients with low levels of cathepsin D and positive nodes actually outlived those with negative nodes and high levels of cathepsin D.

p53

This is the product of a nuclear oncogene and is coded on the short arm of chromosome 17. It appears to be responsible for preventing cellular division in an uncontrolled fashion. As such it works by stabilizing the cell and abnormalities might be expected to allow uncontrolled growth. The protein occurs both as a wild type and as a mutant. Care has to be taken in using an appropriate antibody as the protein is unstable. It seems that a group of patients who have a greatly increased risk of breast, ovarian and bowel cancer (the Li-Fraumeni syndrome) have an abnormality of their p53 expression.

Other factors

Heat shock protein, the antimetastatic gene nm23, p82, laminin receptors, IGF-I receptors and somatostatin receptors are amongst other factors studied. They are not yet in common usage.

Future markers

Molecular biological techniques have expanded the possibilities for more detailed descriptions of individual tumours. Analysis by FISH (fluorescent *in situ* hybridization) will allow 15–20 molecular markers to be simultaneously measured and a phenotypic description provided.

Use of prognostic factors

Patients can be categorized into good or bad prognostic groups on the results of the above factors. They allow definition of a subgroup of node-negative patients whose outlook is so good that no further (adjuvant) treatment is needed and a group of node-positive, high-risk patients whose prognosis is so poor that intensive measures such as high-dose chemotherapy and bone marrow transplantation might be considered. It is rare that anyone has all the characteristics of the good or bad group and the relative merits of each factor needs to be considered before deciding what treatment is appropriate.

DIAGNOSIS OF BREAST CANCER

The majority of patients with breast cancer still present with a breast lump, although it is hoped that the number of patients with impalpable cancers will increase as the Screening Programme should permit earlier identification of breast cancers in the numerically important 50–65-year-old age group. A definite diagnosis should be made on all breast lumps and it should not be assumed that a lump is benign because the mammography or cytology are inconclusive. All patients should have a tissue diagnosis prior to proceeding to definite surgery. This is increasingly made by cytology rather than open biopsy although the latter may still be necessary on occasions. The combination of clinical examination, mammography and fine needle cytology (the triple approach) allows a definitive diagnosis to be made and a treatment plan to be formulated.

If the patient attends a specialist breast clinic the diagnosis may well be established at the time of their first visit. This has considerable advantages in that the news can be broken without a long wait and treatments can be discussed. It is appropriate to have a breast nurse specialist/counsellor present when the diagnosis is given as she will be able to reiterate and reinforce the information passed to the patient as well as acting as a channel for support. A date for staging, surgery (or other primary therapy) can be planned and arrangements for a home visit made. A planned delay of 5–10 days from diagnosis to treatment is often helpful to the patient and her relatives, and allows for the home visit (unfortunately not widely available as yet) or further discussions as appropriate.

Patients referred from the screening service may have a diagnosis of malignancy made on cytology, either by needling of a suspicious area or by stereolocalization of an impalpable lesion. They often need extra care and counselling as they were essentially well women until they attended for mammography. These women are often more anxious by the time they are assessed despite the probability that any lesion picked up at screening is likely to be of better prognosis.

Staging

Once a breast cancer has been diagnosed the patient is staged. The general staging classifications for cancers are not particularly well suited for breast cancer but, as there is no agreement on a better one, the Tumour size-Node-Metastasis (TNM) classification is used. The older UICC stagings are also still in usage but the modern classification of staging and the correlation with TNM is given in Table 6.2.

Table 6.2   TNM classification and relationship to stage

T_{1s}	*in situ*
T_1	<2 cm (T_{1a} ≤ 0.5 cm, T_{1b} >0.5–1.0 cm, T_{1c} >1–2.0 cm)
T_2	>2–5 cm
T_3	>5 cm
T_{4a}	Involvement of chest wall
T_{4b}	Involvement of skin (includes ulceration, direct infiltration, peau d'orange and satellite nodules)
T_{4c}	a and b together
T_{4d}	inflammatory cancer
N_0	No regional node metastasis
N_1	Mobile ipsilateral nodes
N_2	Fixed ipsilateral nodes
N_3	Internal mammary node involvement (rarely clinically detectable)
M_0	No evidence of metastasis
M_1	Distant metastasis (includes ipsilateral supraclavicular nodes)

Correlation of UICC (1987) stage and TNM
Stage I   = T_1, N_0, M_0
Stage II = T_1, N_1, M_0
                    T_2, N_{0-1}, M_0
Stage III =   any T, N_2 or T_3, N_1, M_0 or
                    T_4, N_{0-2}, M_0
Stage IV =   any T, any N, M_1

There is confusion between clinical and pathological staging — tumour size and nodal status often change when the definitive histological report is available. The TNM system was designed to be used clinically and should be reserved for this.

There is a low incidence of detectable metastatic disease in patients with stage I (T_1, N_0) and stage II (T_1, N_1 or T_2, $N_{0,1}$) and, in the absence of hepatomegaly or bone pain, scans of liver and bone have been shown to be worthless. These patients have traditionally had a full blood count, liver function tests and chest X-ray although in younger, fitter patients these investigations are not usually required. For those with bigger or more advanced tumours, bone and liver scans may be ordered if their outcome is going to change clinical management (Table 6.3). Studies have demonstrated that whole body MRI can detect metastases in significant numbers of patients who otherwise are considered as M_0. Studies of the use of MRI as a single screening modality for metastatic disease in patients with apparently localized disease are underway.

The use of tumour markers such as carcinoembryonic antigen (CEA) measurement either alone or in combination with erythrocyte sedimentation rate (ESR) and CA-125 has been advocated by

Table 6.3 Use of staging investigations

Stage	Investigation
I	Full blood count
	Liver function tests
	Chest X-ray
II	As above but may need liver or bone scan if in clinical trials
III	As above but with calcium, phosphate measurement, liver and bone scans
IV	As stage III

some but has low specificity and sensitivity. They may have a place in the follow up of advanced disease.

Once the patient has been staged, decisions have to be made about appropriate therapy. The alternatives should be discussed with the patient and they should be encouraged to participate in decisions. One tool we have found useful in talking through the biology of breast cancer with our patients is to compare breast cancer to a dog. Depending on the stage or prognostic factors, the patient can then be placed on a scale that ranges from a Rottweiler (i.e. a 5 cm Bloom and Richardson grade III lesion with more than 10 nodes positive) to a poodle (0.8 cm screen-detected node-negative tubular cancer) (Fig. 6.4). This allows the patient and relatives to visualize their disease — it obviously works as many patients ask if theirs was a Rottweiler when the results are being discussed. Other methods of helping patients to come to terms with their diagnosis include taping the 'bad

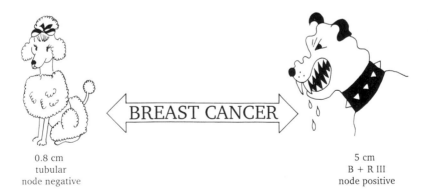

0.8 cm
tubular
node negative

5 cm
B + R III
node positive

Fig. 6.4 A cartoon of an explanation of the biology of breast cancers. Comparing breast cancer to a dog allows visualization of a range of behaviours. B + R III = Bloom and Richardson Grade III carcinoma.

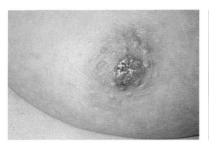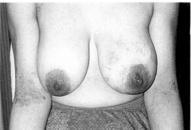

Fig. 2.3 (a) Paget's disease of the nipple; (b) eczema of the nipple.

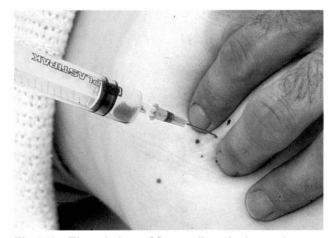

Fig. 2.13 The technique of fine needle aspiration cytology.

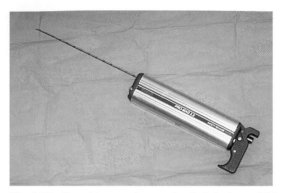

Fig. 2.15 Core biopsy using mechanical device and 14g needle.

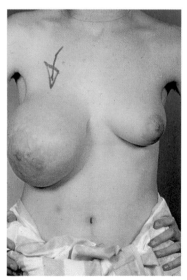

Fig. 3.1 A giant fibroadenoma prior to being removed.

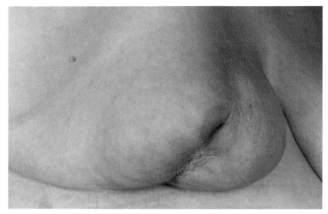

Fig. 3.8   Fat necrosis after a seat belt injury.

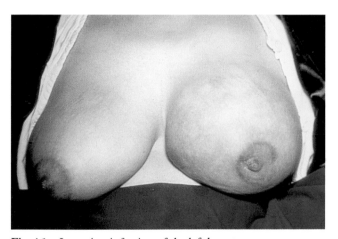

Fig. 4.1   Lactating infection of the left breast.

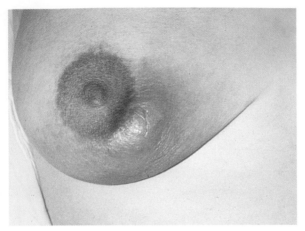

Fig. 4.2   Lactating infection of the right breast.

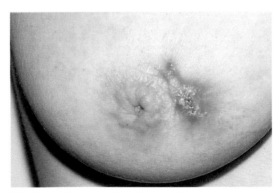

Fig. 4.3   Mammary duct fistula of the right breast.

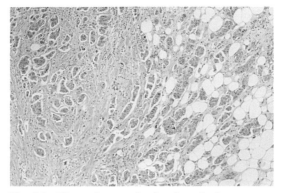

Fig. 6.1 Photomicrograph of an invasive breast cancer.

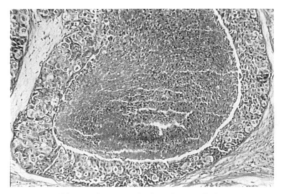

Fig. 6.5 Photomicrograph showing DCIS.

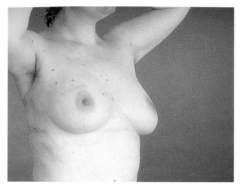

Fig. 6.7 Latissimus dorsi (LD) mini-flap to fill defect after wide local excision of a breast cancer.

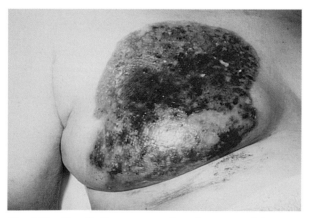

Fig. 6.12 Paget's disease occupying a large area of the breast.

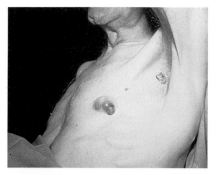

Fig. 6.13 Carcinoma of the male breast. Infiltration of the skin can be seen. The black mark on the skin of the axilla is directly over a palpable and obviously involved axillary node.

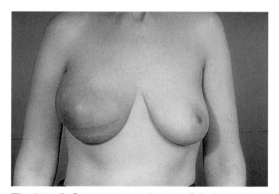

Fig. 7.1 Inflammatory carcinoma of the breast.

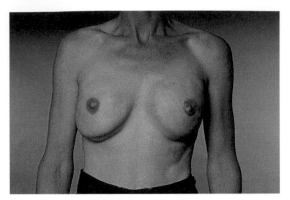

Fig. 8.4 Results of bilateral subcutaneous mastectomy with immediate reconstruction.

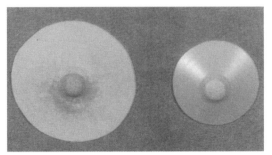

Fig. 8.5 A customized false nipple compared to a commercially obtained one. (Reproduced with permission from Sainsbury et al 1991 Ann Roy Coll Surg Engl 73: 67-69.)

news' consultation and giving the patient the tape to take home. This subject is discussed further in Section 4.

DELAY IN THE DIAGNOSIS OF BREAST CANCER

If screening is effective then it might be argued that diagnosis at the earliest possible stage should lead to improved survival. Conversely, delay in diagnosis should be associated with worse prognosis. Considerable medico-legal interest surrounds this area. Delay may be due to the patient not reporting their symptoms, to the GP not referring appropriately or to the hospital not investigating or missing a diagnosis. When a delay becomes significant is uncertain. For a patient to successfully sue their medical carers they have to prove both that the standard of care fell below the standard that was prevalent at the time they were treated *and* that this led to a less than satisfactory outcome (a loss of chance of survival or a requirement for additional treatments that might not have been required had the cancer been detected earlier). The latter concept of causation is difficult for the medical profession to comprehend as they are trained in a scientific rather than a legal framework.

Complaints and subsequent legal action are on the increase, especially now lawyers are using the contingency fee system. There are several lessons to be learned:

- The patient should always be examined and accurate notes and a diagram made.
- The national guidelines on referral should be followed.
- A solid discrete lump must have a definite diagnosis — if this cannot be obtained by triple assessment then the lump should be removed.
- Beware a lumpy area that doesn't feel right and images as normal breast tissue.
- Invasive lobular cancer typically presents as diffuse disease with symptoms that do not match the signs.
- A typical breast cancer is easy to diagnose — it is the atypical one in a young patient that causes diagnostic problems.

TREATMENT OF BREAST CANCER

Introduction

Discussions of the management of breast cancer traditionally divide the subject into early and advanced categories. This was based on the criteria of operability with 'early' usually encompassing stages I and II and advanced being stages III and IV disease. The use of 'early' is a misnomer as true early breast cancer would be too small to detect clinically as, once a tumour is palpable, micrometastatic disease is probable. Early should refer to the biology of the tumour. Some patients present with large ulcerated cancers that have been present for a long time and yet they have no evidence of metastases whilst some present with metastatic disease with a very small primary (and some without a detectable lesion at all).

The treatment of the patient with 'early' breast cancer has two main aims — to achieve local disease control and to treat any micrometastatic disease. Although breast cancer is often a systemic disease at presentation, there are many patients who are cured by primary surgery (with or without radiotherapy) alone. Deciding which patients need further therapy has recently been simplified but many questions remain to be answered.

Treatment of non-invasive breast cancer

Ductal carcinoma in situ (DCIS)

Reports of the natural history of DCIS are based on the review of biopsies performed many years earlier which were classified by their original pathologist as benign, a few of which, on review, were classified as having areas of DCIS (Fig. 6.5). A recent updated study from Nashville, USA of 28 patients with DCIS undiagnosed on biopsy, reports that by 30 years, 40% had developed an invasive breast cancer all at the original biopsy site. The 40% who developed breast cancer were thought to belong to the group where it was estimated that the biopsy did not remove all DCIS. A second study from New York reported similar rates of cancer development. All lesions in Nashville and New York series were low grade. A third study of 80 patients included two patients with high-grade DCIS and a significant number of patients with lesions that others call atypical ductal hyperplasia. After a mean follow up of 17.5 years, 20% in this series had developed invasive cancer or recurrent DCIS. From these data it appears that following an incomplete excision, between 20% and 60% of patients with low-grade DCIS lesions will develop recurrent DCIS or an invasive cancer at the same site in the breast over a 20-year period, with the majority of these developing in the first decade. There is little information on the behaviour of inadequately excised intermediate and high-grade DCIS, although there is a suspicion that recurrence may occur more often. It is exemplified by an 80%

recurrence rate at 5 years reported in one series in patients with high-grade DCIS treated by wide excision alone.

Initially, all DCIS was treated by mastectomy and this treatment produces between 98% and 99% cause-specific survival at 10 years. The identification of small areas of DCIS by screening and the use of breast conservation for invasive cancers has resulted in an increasing trend away from mastectomy towards breast conservation for DCIS. Although a small percentage of DCIS lesions are currently managed by mastectomy, as a result of increasing incidence, the actual number of patients with DCIS treated by mastectomy rose in the USA from 3478 in 1983 to 4200 in 1992. Some treat localized DCIS by wide local excision alone, whereas others give routine radiotherapy after adequate excision with a few selecting treatment on the basis of type or extent of DCIS. The predominant view has been to treat the whole breast, whether by mastectomy or radiotherapy.

Treating all DCIS lesions in the same manner makes little sense as studies have shown marked biological and behavioural differences between histological types of DCIS. Biological differences include differences in oncogene expression, with 80% of high-grade DCIS staining positive for the oncogene erbB2, whereas only 10% of low-grade DCIS expressed erbB2; the same is true for the tumour suppressor gene p53 with over 60% of high-grade, but less than 5% of low-grade lesions, demonstrating over-expression. The presence of significant amounts of ER also differs between histological subtypes with 28% of comedo DCIS being ER positive compared with 50% in non-comedo DCIS.

The variable behaviour of different histological types of DCIS is manifested by a much higher recurrence rate after breast conservation in patients whose DCIS is high grade or contains areas of moderate or marked necrosis. In contrast, there are very few instances where recurrence occurred after complete excision of low-grade DCIS. There may also be differences in the effectiveness of radiotherapy in preventing local recurrence followed by local excision in different histological types of DCIS. Recently updated data from the National Surgical Adjuvant Breast Project (NSABP) demonstrated in the group treated by wide excision alone, that 26% developed local recurrence after a median follow up of 8 years — a figure very similar to that seen when invasive cancer is treated by excision alone. In this study, radiotherapy reduced *in situ* recurrence by approximately 42% and invasive recurrence by approximately 69%, and appeared to be of particular benefit in reducing recurrence in lesions with a marked or moderate necrosis. This is consistent with an earlier study which reported that radiotherapy significantly reduced the recurrence rate in high-grade, but not other types of DCIS.

The role of tamoxifen in DCIS is unclear and it is being investigated in the current UK DCIS trial. Assuming approximately two-thirds of ER positive lesions gain some benefit from an agent such as tamoxifen, one can estimate that 19% of comedo and 34% of noncomedo DCIS are likely to be influenced by this treatment. This view is supported by the findings in a model system — tamoxifen fails to reduce epithelial proliferation of comedo type DCIS. Current scientific knowledge suggests therefore that tamoxifen will have little impact on the behaviour of comedo DCIS. A contralateral breast cancer appears at a similar annual rate in patients with either DCIS or an invasive breast cancer and therefore tamoxifen may still have a role in DCIS by reducing contralateral disease development.

As trends to treat DCIS by breast conservation increase, it is important to know which factors predict for local recurrence after wide local excision. Apart from histological type, extent of DCIS and completeness of excision appear important. Studies of mastectomies performed for DCIS have suggested that lesions over 4 cm are unlikely to be adequately excised by wide local excision or quadrantectomy and this is supported by the high local recurrence rates reported following breast-conserving therapy for lesions over 4 cm. Completeness of excision can be difficult to define for the pathologist although it is possible to measure the distance of normal tissue to the nearest lateral margin. New data show that as the width of normal tissue removed increases, so the risk of local recurrence appears to decrease. By scoring the three major predictors for recurrence — histological type, disease extent and width of normal tissue excised around the DCIS — a prognostic index has been developed to help select the most appropriate treatment for individual patients. By adding the scores derived from these three important factors, groups of patients have been identified who might best be treated by wide local excision alone, wide local excision and radiotherapy, or mastectomy (Table 6.4). This approach is open to a number of criticisms, not least of which is that the index needs to be confirmed in another data set before the results can be considered for clinical use. There is also doubt whether the simple addition of factors will provide clear solutions as to how this complex and variable disease should be managed. Nonetheless these data and those from the NSABP indicate that a significant number of patients are likely to benefit from post-operative radiotherapy. The important, and at present unanswered, question is exactly which are these

Table 6.4   Van Nuys prognostic index for DCIS

	Score		
	1	2	3
Disease extent			
● >15 mm	x		
● 15–40 mm		x	
● <40 mm			x
Margin			
● <10 mm	x		
● 1–9 mm		x	
● 1 mm			x
Histological type			
● Non-high grade	x		
● High grade, no necrosis		x	
● High grade + necrosis			x

It is suggested that patients with a score of 3, 4 and 5 be treated by wide local excision, 6 and 7 by wide local excision and radiotherapy, and 8 and 9 by mastectomy.

patients? A guide for DCIS management is outline in Table 6.5. If a mastectomy is performed, it is usual to sample lower axillary nodes as between 1% and 5% of patients with DCIS do have positive nodes. An axillary clearance should never be performed.

Lobular carcinoma in situ (LCIS)

This rarer form of non-invasive breast cancer differs in presentation, biological behaviour and implications for treatment. LCIS does not typically form microcalcifications and is therefore not eas-

Table 6.5   Recommended treatment for ductal carcinoma *in situ**

Localised carcinoma in situ *(<4 cm)§*
● Wide local excision
   Ensure that mammographic lesion has been completely excised with clear histological margins
   Re-excise if margins are involved
   Consider mastectomy if carcinoma >4 cm in size or if micropapillary
● Consider post-operative radiotherapy if high grade + necrosis/comedo type DCIS
● Consider tamoxifen, 20 mg a day if ER positive

Widespread carcinoma in situ *(≥4 cm)§*
● Mastectomy (with or without breast reconstruction)
● Consider tamoxifen if ER positive

*Outside clinical trials
§Extent of carcinoma can be estimated in 80% of patients by measuring extent of malignant microcalcification on mammograms

ily detectable on X-ray, and is usually found incidentally on biopsy. It can be found in the contralateral breast in 30% of cases and in the residual breast (if treated by mastectomy) in up to 70% of cases. If LCIS is associated with invasive lobular carcinoma, the incidence of nodal involvement is very low and LCIS having been diagnosed by biopsy should be treated by careful follow up in the expectation of ipsilateral or contralateral disease which may be invasive. This should take the form of clinical examination, annual mammography with ultrasound and biopsy of any area of suspicion. Many would now regard LCIS as a marker of subsequent breast cancer rather than as a premalignant lesion.

Treatment of invasive breast cancer

Local control

Local control is important. A recurrence in the mastectomy wound or at the site of a local resection is damaging both oncologically and psychologically. There is debate about whether such a recurrence compromises survival (the majority of reports claim that it does not) but it does require further treatment. The adoption of more conservative surgery might be expected to lead to a higher incidence of recurrence, but this can be minimized by achieving clear resection margins and by the subsequent use of radiotherapy. In addition, patients with large, aggressive tumours should be advised to consider mastectomy.

Conservation therapy

Not everyone is suitable for conservation therapy — those with multifocal disease on clinical examination or mammography or a large, centrally placed tumour are often better off with a mastectomy as the resultant defect is not attractive and it may be impossible to provide a satisfactory prosthesis. These patients can be offered a reconstruction either as a primary or secondary procedure. In some centres primary systemic therapy, usually chemotherapy, is offered to those with large tumours to downstage them and thus allow smaller resections (known as primary medical or neoadjuvant therapy).

The aim of achieving local control includes attention to the axilla. There is still a great deal of debate about how the axilla should be managed, and this is addressed later.

Local control is achieved by the use of surgery in the majority of cases (because most patients are still referred to surgeons and because it is often an appropriate modality).

Whilst it is possible to treat even small cancers with chemotherapy and radiotherapy, this is time consuming and tends to be reserved for large T_2, T_3 and T_4 lesions. Large doses of radiotherapy are needed in the presence of an intact tumour and cosmesis is, generally, poor. For smaller cancers breast conservation is the most common primary treatment. This takes the form of a wide local excision performed through an appropriate incision to give a good cosmetic result (see Fig. 6.6).

Impalpable lesions should be investigated by stereotactic or ultrasound-guided fine needle aspiration cytology (FNAC) as appropriate and Figure 2.19 outlines how this assists in the management of these patients. In units without access to stereotactic aspiration cytology, patients with lesions considered to be suspicious should have these either widely excised or biopsied depending on the degree of suspicion, with any lymph node surgery being performed as a separate procedure.

Patients suitable for breast conservation are listed in Table 6.6 and include:

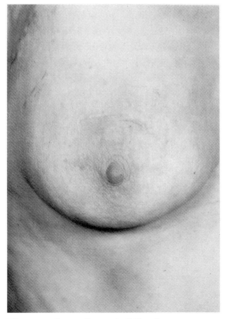

Fig. 6.6 Cosmetic result following conservation therapy.

- Those with a single clinical and mammographic lesion measuring 4 cm or less without signs of local advancement (T_1, T_2 <4 cm), extensive nodal involvement (N_0, N_1) or metastases (M_0).
- Those with tumours bigger than 4 cm and large breasts.

There is no age limit for breast conservation and elderly, fit patients should be treated in the same way as younger patients.

Lesions which are potentially unsuitable for breast conservation are summarized in Table 6.6 and include:

- Patients for whom breast conservation treatment would produce an unacceptable cosmetic result. This includes the majority of central lesions and carcinomas over 4 cm in size; additionally, these larger tumours have been excluded from most prospective studies of breast conservation and so there is little information on the outcome of treating such tumours by conservation. Having said this, size is not a factor in relation to local recurrence so the only reason these larger tumours have not been traditionally treated by conservation is because of the cosmetic outcome. It is now possible to treat large unifocal breast cancers that previously would have required a mastectomy by a wide excision, filling the defect left after the wide excision by the latissimus dorsi muscle with overlying fat. The role of this mini-flap is under evaluation in some centres but produces excellent cosmetic results and allows increasing numbers of patients to be treated by conservation. It has the advantage, compared with primary systemic therapy, that the nodal status is known at the outset and so appropriate systemic therapy can be instituted after wide excision. Because of the importance of obtaining clear margins in breast conservation, these mini-flap procedures are often performed in two stages. The

Table 6.6 Indications and contraindications for selection of patients for breast conservation (adapted from NIH Consensus Conference Statement 1991)

Indications	T_1, T_2, ($\leq$4 cm), N_0, N_1, M_0
	T_2 >4 cm in large breasts
Contraindications	T_3–T_4, N_2 or M_1
	Large or central tumours in small breasts
	Multifocal/multicentric disease
	Collagen vascular disease
Relative contraindications	An extensive *in situ* component
	Young age (under 35–39 years)
	Widespread lymphatic invasion

first stage is a very wide excision and the second stage a level III axillary clearance combined with a latissimus dorsi mini-flap (Fig. 6.7). This ensures that patients have clear margins at the time of flap reconstruction.

Radiotherapy can safely be given to the whole breast to ensure local recurrence is kept to the same levels that would be expected after standard treatment. A boost to the tumour resection site is usually omitted. It is also possible to shrink large tumours using primary medical therapy and thus allowing breast-conserving surgery to be performed. In Milan, tumours measuring 3 cm or over were traditionally treated by mastectomy, but in a series of over 150 of these tumours, treated by primary chemotherapy, 81% were reduced in size to less than 3 cm and were subsequently suitable for treatment by breast conservation.

- Patients with multiple macroscopic tumour foci treated by breast conservation have a high incidence of local recurrence and are better treated by mastectomy, ideally with immediate breast reconstruction. Although multifocal or multicentric disease may be evident clinically, it is often only identified by mammography.
- Patients with bilateral disease can be treated by bilateral conservation, but bilateral mastectomy with immediate reconstruction is preferred by some.

Certain clinical and pathological factors may also influence selection of patients for breast conservation, because of their potential impact on local recurrence after breast-conserving therapy. These include young age (<35–39 years), the presence of extensive DCIS associated with the invasive tumour (EIC) and widespread lymphatic invasion.

As clear resection margins are important to reduce local relapse, care should be taken to widely excise the lesion. The edges should be identified by clips or sutures to allow orientation of the specimen. Some surgeons go on to take cavity shavings — this allows the pathologist to confirm if the resection margins are clear. If tumour is present in the shavings, then either further local excision or a mastectomy is indicated. It is clear from the literature that radiotherapy will not always compensate for involved margins. A quadrantectomy (tylectomy) is popular in some countries but is a misnomer in that it is impossible to divide the breast into discrete quadrants. Such excisions aim to get wider margins (3 cm) and are associated with higher rates of local control but much poorer cosmetic outcomes.

Local surgery alone may be sufficient treatment for small areas of DCIS or small invasive tumours of special type. This hypothesis is being tested in a trial run by the British Association of Surgical Oncology (BASO) where patients with special type and well-differentiated cancers are, after surgery, randomized to no further treatment or radiotherapy and/or tamoxifen.

Wide local excision of palpable lesions

The aim of this procedure is to remove the palpable lesion with a 1 cm margin of surrounding normal breast tissue. The incision should either be placed along Langer's lines or the lines of maximum skin crease tension (see Fig. 2.16). It is inappropriate to use circumareolar incisions for lesions some distance away from the nipple because re-excision, if required, is almost impossible through such an incision. Removal of skin overlying the lesion is unnecessary unless the lesion is very superficial. The cosmetic result after breast-conserving surgery is influenced by the amount of skin excised, poor results being obtained in those who have had a large amount of skin removed. If the patient has had a previous incomplete excision, then the previous scar should be excised. Having made the skin incision, the fingers of the left hand are placed over the lesion and dissection is performed 1 cm beyond the fingertips so that the line of incision through the breast tissue is beyond the limit of the carcinoma. Although in superficial lesions it is sometimes necessary to dissect in the plane between the breast tissue and subcutaneous fat, skin flaps should not be undermined by dissecting into this fat, as thin skin flaps are associated with a poor post-operative cosmetic appearance. Dissection is continued through the breast down to the pectoral fascia with no attempt being made to excise this fascia, unless it is tethered to the tumour or the tumour is directly involving it. Where the carcinoma infiltrates the muscle, a fillet of muscle should be removed, the aim being to gain a rim of normal tissue around the tumour. Having reached the pectoral fascia, the breast is elevated from this fascia, the lesion grasped between fingers and thumb and excision completed at the other margins. In superficial lesions, an adequate excision can usually be performed without excising a full thickness portion of breast tissue down to pectoral fascia. Specimens should be orientated prior to submission to a pathologist with sutures or ligaclips. Meticulous haemostasis is secured with diathermy, the cavity can be lavaged with diluted savlon left *in situ* for 2 min. Savlon (dilute chlorhexadine) has been shown to be tumoricidal at this concentration and within this time period.

Stereotactic wide local excision

Impalpable lesions are localized prior to surgery (Fig. 6.8) as discussed earlier for needle localization biopsy. Using the mammograms as a guide, a block of tissue 1–2 cm around the mammographic lesion is excised. The specimen is orientated with ligaclips and then X-rayed (Fig. 6.9). The radiograph of the excised specimen is inspected during the operation and, having orientated the specimen with ligaclips, it is possible to assess the completeness of excision; if the lesion approaches any resection margin, further tissue can be excised and orientated from the appropriate area. Using this technique it is possible to achieve complete excision in over 80% of both invasive and *in situ* carcinomas. Wound management after the lesion has been excised is as for wide local excision.

Post-operative radiotherapy

Radiotherapy services are provided on a regional or sub-regional basis and patients may have to travel long distances for this treatment. Commonly the radiation is given using a linear accelerator to deliver high energy X-rays with 40–50 Gy (equivalent to 4000–5000 rad) being given to the breast over 4 weeks in daily fractions of 180–200 cGY. Some centres prescribe higher doses and the dose per

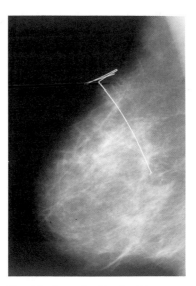

Fig. 6.8   Stereolocalization biopsy with needle passing through abnormal area to be excised.

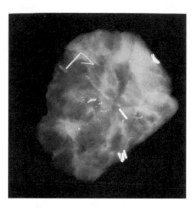

Fig. 6.9   Specimen X-ray following excision with marking clips.

fraction may also vary. A top-up or boost (15–20 Gy) to the excision site can be given by further external beam irradiation or by the use of radioactive implants. These are typically iridium wires which are inserted around the tumour site. Precise indications for boosting and techniques are not well defined.

The survival rates after lumpectomy are equivalent to those after more radical surgery, and the former is now the treatment of choice for appropriate patients. The swing away from mastectomy as the routine operation for patients with breast cancer is to be welcomed but must not become a goal in its own right — the interests of some patients will be compromised if the only operation offered is a lumpectomy.

The axilla will be irradiated if it has not been treated by surgery and the ipsilateral supraclavicular fossa may also be treated if the axillary nodes were involved. The addition of radiotherapy to lumpectomy reduced the local recurrence rate from 39% to 10% in the National Surgical Adjuvant Breast Project B-06 (NSABP B-06) (see Chapter 9) and reductions from 25% to 5% are quoted in other studies.

Risk factors for local recurrence after breast conservation

Large variations have been reported (2–22% at 5 years) from different centres in rates of recurrence within the treated breast following breast-conservation therapy for invasive breast carcinoma.

Patient-related factors

Rates of local recurrence appear to correlate closely with age, being more frequent in younger patients. In women under the age of 35 the risk of local recurrence is approximately three times the risk of patients over the age of 50 (Table 6.7). A single study has indicated that breast recurrence is less frequent in women with large breasts, whether this relates to it being possible to perform more generous excisions in these patients is unknown.

Tumour-related factors

Tumour location, size, the presence of skin or nipple retraction and the presence or absence of axillary nodal involvement have not been consistently shown to be factors predictive of recurrence within the breast following conservation therapy. Local failure rates appear to relate to:

The completeness of excision. If the pathologist reports the presence of invasive or *in situ* cancer at the margins of the excision, then local recurrence is approximately four times more likely to occur than if the margins are reported to be clear.

The presence of an extensive in situ component (EIC). If 25% of the tumour mass is composed of *in situ* carcinoma, and *in situ* carcinoma is also present in the tissue surrounding the tumour, then the carcinoma is considered to have an EIC. Patients who have a tumour which is EIC positive have approximately three times the risk of local recurrence compared to patients whose tumours are EIC negative. When one studies the interaction between margins and EIC, margins appear to be more important than EIC. Two studies have shown that patients who had clear margins in the presence of an extensive *in situ* component had very low rates of local recurrence whereas in those whose tumour had EIC and involved margins rates of local recurrence were unacceptable. In the presence of EIC, it is therefore absolutely essential that patients have a complete excision.

Lymphatic/vascular invasion. If the pathologist reports the presence of tumour within vascular or lymphatic channels within or around the invasive cancer, then breast recurrence is approximately twice as common as tumours where this feature is absent.

Table 6.7   Relationships between age and local recurrence rates at 5 years following breast-conserving treatment

Age	Local recurrence rate
<35	17%
35–50	12%
>51	6%

Histological grade. Patients with low-grade tumours appear to be at low risk of local recurrence. There appears to be a stepwise increase in local recurrence as the grade increases although not all studies have shown major differences in local recurrence between tumours of histological grade II and III.

Treatment-related factors

As outlined above, the completeness of excision is a major factor predicting local recurrence. Both the completeness of excision and the amount of normal tissue removed around the carcinoma appear to be related to local disease control — the wider the margins the lower the rate of local recurrence. The volume of normal tissue excised is particularly important in tumours which are EIC positive. In these cancers a very wide excision is necessary to gain adequate local control rates.

Radiotherapy, chemotherapy and tamoxifen all reduce local relapse rates after breast-conserving therapy. Radiotherapy is routinely used as part of breast-conserving therapy because of the clear reduction in local recurrence rates. The interval between surgery and radiotherapy may be important and there are suggestions that the rate of local recurrence increases if radiotherapy is delayed. There is some evidence to suggest that increased doses of radiotherapy improve local control rates, but the higher the dose of radiotherapy given, the poorer the overall cosmetic result. There is thus a delicate balance between achieving adequate local control rates and satisfactory cosmetic results (Fig. 6.6).

Significance and treatment of local recurrence

An isolated breast recurrence does not appear to be a threat to survival, although breast recurrence is a predictor of distant disease which should be sought in all patients presenting with an apparently isolated breast recurrence. Isolated recurrences can be treated by re-excision or mastectomy. Although it is known that re-excision is associated with a high rate of further recurrence, if the initial recurrence occurs more than 5 years after surgery and the margins of the re-excision are clear of disease, adequate long-term control can be achieved. For local recurrences not fulfilling these criteria, mastectomy is indicated unless the local recurrence is associated with metastatic disease when systemic therapy is required. Uncontrollable local recurrence is uncommon after breast conservation but does occur and is difficult to treat.

Diagnosis of a recurrence after previous local excision and radiotherapy is not always straightforward and there may be a delay in achieving a diagnosis. Cytology can be misleading and mammography difficult to interpret. MRI appears to be the diagnostic imaging test of choice in this situation.

The criteria for conservation therapy are shown in Table 6.6.

PRIMARY MEDICAL THERAPY

This is increasingly being used for larger operable breast cancers. Induction (neoadjuvant) chemotherapy has been shown to shrink large T_2 and T_3 tumours and thus allow quadrantectomy rather than mastectomy. Figure 6.10 shows the mammograms of a patient with a large breast cancer receiving combination chemotherapy. The tumour mass can clearly be seen to have disappeared although the microcalcifications remain. Failure to proceed to some form of additional treatment (usually surgery) will lead to local relapse. It seems likely that even patients with a complete clinical response cannot be managed by radiotherapy alone but require surgery. The surgery may be difficult as there may be little to feel on dissection and a localizing wire may be necessary. Post-operative consolidation chemotherapy is usually given (Fig. 6.11).

MASTECTOMY

Historically, mastectomy has been the treatment of choice for breast cancer as the prevalent hypothesis was of a centrifugal spread of

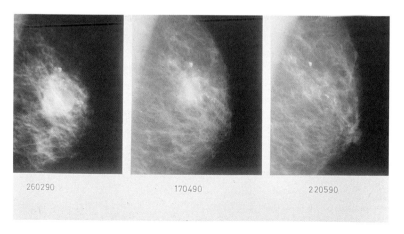

260290   170490   220590

Fig. 6.10   Three mammograms from a patient undergoing primary medical treatment showing disappearance of the tumour mass. Note that the microcalcifications remain.

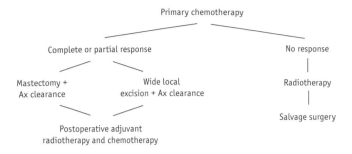

Fig. 6.11 Primary medical therapy to downstage large carcinomas.

breast cancer cells. The lymph nodes were supposed to act as filters with secondary spread occurring only when their capacity was exhausted. It therefore seemed logical to perform ever more 'heroic' (extensive) surgery in an attempt to get beyond the growing edge of the tumour. This dogma, based on the studies of Handley, held sway for 100 years and was championed by Halsted whose name is still attached to a radical mastectomy. In the 1920s some American surgeons went so far as to perform forequarter amputations in an attempt to clear the disease.

A mastectomy is now taken to be an operation that removes the breast tissue with some overlying skin (including the nipple). This is termed a total mastectomy. If the skin and nipple are left intact and the breast tissue removed, the operation is termed a subcutaneous mastectomy. A radical mastectomy includes removal of the pectoralis muscles and the axillary contents. This was modified by Patey (modified radical mastectomy) who left the pectoralis major muscle but divided pectoralis minor which still allowed the axilla to be cleared. The most common breast resection operation in this country is a total mastectomy combined with a limited axillary dissection or sampling ('simple mastectomy') or with a full axillary clearance ('modified radical mastectomy').

Technique

The incisions are planned to allow skin flaps to be created which will close neatly but without undue tension. They should be of equal length to prevent 'dog ears' in the final scar. Dissection is performed under the flaps until the fascia covering the pectoralis muscles is reached. Breast tissue is then elevated from the fascia and removed. Haemostasis is achieved with ties or diathermy, and low pressure suction drains are inserted under the skin to remove serosanguinous exudate and to allow the flaps to stick to the chest wall. The wound is closed with subcutaneous and subcuticular sutures such as polydioxone sulphate (Ethicon) or Maxon (Davis and Geck). No formal dressing is required although Steri-strips applied to the length of the wound and then crossways across it reduce any wound edge oedema and give a neater final scar. The patient begins arm exercises, taught preoperatively, on the day after surgery and the drains are removed when the drainage is less then 50 ml. The length of time they drain depends on the extent of axillary surgery.

Complications after mastectomy

These include seroma, infection and flap necrosis.

Seroma

These occur in the dead space under the flaps and are caused by the transudation of fluid across the large surface area where the breast and lymphatics once were. Suction drainage has been shown in several trials to be effective in reducing significant seromas as well as reducing the incidence of wound infection. They should be of low pressure as high pressure suction merely collapses skin around the drain and blocks it.

Infection

This is generally secondary to tissue necrosis caused by cutting the flaps too thin which results in devascularization. Prophylactic antibiotics are not indicated unless for some other underlying reason such as the insertion of a tissue expander or prostheses — good surgical technique is more important.

Flap necrosis

Again this is usually as a result of technical shortcomings secondary to devascularization of the flaps.

Other complications

These are rare but include pneumothorax and injury to neurovascular structures.

Radiotherapy after mastectomy

The question of whether chest wall irradiation is indicated after mastectomy was controversial, but its role has been better defined. Studies by McWhirter in Edinburgh showed that simple mastectomy and radiotherapy was as effective a treatment as radical mastectomy in terms of both disease control and survival. The more recent Cancer Research Campaign (CRC) trial, where 2800 women with stage I and II breast cancer were randomized to receive radiotherapy or no radiotherapy after mastectomy, showed no difference in survival but demonstrated a marked improvement in local control rates for those receiving radiotherapy. Those not having radiotherapy had approximately three times the risk of local recurrence, the majority of which (but not all) were controllable by radiotherapy given at the time of relapse. At one time radiotherapy was standard treatment after all mastectomies but there is now a more selective policy. The indications for radiotherapy postmastectomy are:

- Large tumours (>4 cm).
- High-grade tumours (Bloom and Richardson grade III).
- Node-positive tumours (>4), especially if extranodal disease is seen.
- Node-negative tumours with widespread vascular/lymphatic invasion.

Two recent papers have shown a survival advantage for patients who are at high risk because of involved nodes who receive radiotherapy. Those in the remaining group who go on to develop local recurrence can be treated at that time in the knowledge that, in the majority, disease will be controlled by this treatment.

An excess of cardiac deaths was seen in patients with left-sided cancers treated with orthovoltage radiotherapy machines due to irradiation of the left anterior descending coronary artery. Such an effect is no longer seen with modern machines and planning techniques that reduce coronary artery irradiation.

THE AXILLA

Introduction

This subject, more than any other, still causes heated debate. The options for axillary treatment range from nothing through sampling and limited axillary dissection, with or without subsequent radiotherapy, to formal clearance. The combination of a complete axillary clearance with radiotherapy causes unacceptable arm oedema and is now avoided.

The major lymphatic drainage of the breast is to the axilla and the axillary nodes are divided into three levels (Fig. 1.5).

There are, on average, 13.5 lymph nodes present at level I, 4.5 nodes at level II and 2.3 nodes at level III. Very few patients have lymph nodes involved at level II or level III in the absence of level I involvement. These so-called skip metastases occurred in only 1.3% of patients who were axillary node positive in a large series published from Milan.

Axillary node status remains the single best prognostic factor and important treatment decisions are based upon it. In addition, the axilla needs treatment to prevent uncontrolled local disease. This can be provided either by surgery or radiotherapy, although using the latter without knowing if the nodes contain tumour means that some people will receive radiotherapy unnecessarily.

How much surgery and for whom is also controversial. Clinical examination of the axilla correlates badly with true nodal status as assessed histologically; some form of sampling is therefore needed. There are, as yet, no good imaging techniques for the axilla and this is one area where a major advance is needed. (Early reports on the use of MRI sound promising.)

Role of axillary surgery

The role of axillary surgery is twofold:

- To stage the axilla.
- To treat axillary disease.

Non-operative techniques of staging the axilla including clinical examination and various radiological techniques are unsatisfactory. Surgical options which have been described in the axilla have included: a single-node biopsy, initially blind but more recently guided by scintigraphy or a vital dye; an axillary node sample — removing four nodes from the axilla; axillary dissection to a landmark such as the intercostobrachial nerve; a level I dissection; a level II dissection, and a level III dissection.

Staging of the axilla is also important for selection of adjuvant therapy, providing prognostic information and providing an index of efficacy of screening programmes.

Ability of these procedures to stage the axilla

Sentinel node biopsy is performed by injecting methylene blue or Tc-labelled sulphur colloid (or both) into the skin over the tumour or directly into and around the tumour. Subsequent localization and biopsy of the sentinel node has demonstrated a good relationship between its involvement and axillary nodal status. In a large series, from Milan, excision of the sentinel node alone would have provided an accurate assessment of axillary lymph node status in 97.5% of patients. One problem with this technique is that the node needs to be removed and submitted for histological assessment so there is a time delay. Thus sentinel node biopsy and the axillary dissection, if necessary, cannot be performed at the same time. Frozen section of lymph nodes has been investigated but is associated with approximately a 10% false negative rate.

Much debate has surrounded the use of axillary node sampling. Axillary dissection to a particular landmark (the intercostobrachial nerve being the most commonly used) is inaccurate in assessing whether the patient has involved axillary nodes. Data from Edinburgh on 401 patients undergoing a mastectomy and randomized to either an axillary node sample or an axillary node clearance, showed that the axillary node sample group had a node positivity rate of 42% whereas those undergoing clearance had a node positivity rate of 40%. This suggests that both are equally effective at staging the axilla. This is supported by further data on 135 patients who, having undergone an axillary node sample, were then randomized to have either a clearance or no more surgery. Of the 67 patients who initially underwent sampling and then went on to have a clearance, 41 patients were node negative on the sample; none of these converted to node positive on the clearance.

Using data from Milan, a mathematical model has been formulated to determine the number of nodes which have to be present in a level I sample to have a 90% chance of predicting true node-negative status. This mathematical model suggests that at least 10 nodes have to be sampled. The problem with these data and results from other similar studies are that they presume that all nodes in the axilla are equally likely to be sampled. Data from this mathematical model indicate that when only five nodes are sampled at level I, there would only be a 73% chance of picking up all node-positive patients. If this model were applied to the data from the Edinburgh randomized study, 10 out of 41 patients classified as node negative should have had unrecognized positive nodes. None actually did. This model also predicts that four-node sampling should not be a satisfactory procedure in staging the axilla, and yet clinical data clearly indicate that it is. In node sampling it is the four largest nodes which are sampled which differs from a level I dissection where all axillary fat and lymph nodes are removed within the anatomical boundaries of level I (Fig. 1.5). The mathematical model probably does apply if a formal anatomical level I dissection is performed, in which case a minimum of 10 nodes are needed to be certain that the axillary disease is accurately staged. Axillary dissection to level II or level III is effective at assessing the axillary lymph node status as the majority or all nodes are removed from the axilla. An axillary node sample (four nodes), a level I dissection (10 nodes) or a level II and III clearance will all adequately stage the axilla.

Treatment of axillary disease

There are two main options for treating the involved axilla:

- Radical radiotherapy.
- Full level III axillary clearance.

Even in patients with one node positive at level I, there is a significant chance of nodes at level II or III being involved (Table 6.8); this chance increases as the number of positive nodes at level I increases. A level I dissection alone can, therefore, never be considered a therapeutic procedure in a patient who has even a single axillary nodal metastasis. The same problem arises with a level II dissection in that 50% of those with level II involvement also have disease at level III. A level II dissection thus gives no more information than can be gleaned from an axillary node sample or a level I dissection and does not adequately treat the involved axilla.

Studies of axillary recurrence generally indicate that in patients with involved axillary nodes, axillary clearance provides lower

Table 6.8 Correlation of number of involved axillary nodes at level I with percentage of patients who will have involved nodes at levels II and III

Number positive at level I	% with positive nodes at level II and III
1	12
2	19
3	37
4	40
5	84

recurrence rates than radical radiotherapy (Table 6.9). These differences are, however, not dramatic and a 95% control rate of disease in the axilla at 8 years in patients with involved nodes is possible using radiotherapy.

Morbidity of radiotherapy and axillary clearance

The complications include lymphoedema and damage to nerves in the axilla (surgically this is division of the intercostobrachial, long thoracic or thoracodorsal nerves and with radiotherapy the rare complication of brachial plexopathy). Another problem with radiotherapy is that it can induce sarcomas. The incidence of these complications is summarized in Table 6.10. The aim in the axilla must be to limit morbidity as well as achieve disease control.

There are some who believe that surgeons should not enter the axilla. This group suggests that clinically involved axillae should be treated with radical radiotherapy and, in the remainder, a watch policy should be adopted, treating only those patients who develop symptomatic axillary relapse. Administering radiotherapy to the axillae of all patients with palpable axillary nodes ignores the fact that up to 40% will not have axillary node involvement and will thus be receiving unnecessary treatment which is associated with significant morbidity. Important information in deciding adjuvant treatment and prognosis is also not obtained. The watch policy —

Table 6.9 Control of axillary disease from National Surgical Adjuvant Breast Project Protocol B-04

	Clinically node +ve		Clinically node -ve	
	Mx Cl	**Mx XRT**	**Mx Cl**	**Mx XRT**
% axillary recurrence	1	11.9	1.4	3.1

Mx = mastectomy, Cl = axillary node clearance, XRT = radiotherapy

Table 6.10 Morbidity after axillary procedures

	XRT	**Cl**	**NS**
Lymphoedema	+	+	0
Nerve problems	+	+	0/+
Sarcomas	+	0	0
ROM at shoulder	+/++	+	0/+

XRT = radiotherapy, Cl = axillary clearance, NS = axillary node sample, ROM = range of movement

treating disease only when it becomes clinically evident — is based on the findings of the NSABP B-04 trial, which randomized patients who were clinically axillary node negative to receive a mastectomy and axillary node clearance, mastectomy and radiotherapy, or a mastectomy alone. The results of this study are summarized in Table 6.11. As can be seen, only 18% of those who did not have either full axillary clearance or radiotherapy subsequently developed axillary relapse, and there were no differences between the groups in overall survival at 10 years. There are, however, a number of problems with this study in that one-third of the mastectomy group who apparently received mastectomy alone did have a limited axillary dissection. Although over 20% of patients developed symptomatic axillary disease if no nodes were excised during the mastectomy, this was reduced to 8% if there was a very limited lower axillary dissection, whereas no one had symptomatic disease if more than five nodes were removed as part of the mastectomy. It was also evident that a number of patients in the mastectomy-only group who developed axillary recurrence had uncontrollable axillary disease.

Lymphoedema

This is uncommon after a simple mastectomy and its incidence rises with the amount of axillary surgery performed. The combination of extensive axillary surgery and radiotherapy gives a high incidence of lymphoedema and should be avoided. When it occurs, compression therapy either by means of a mechanical sleeve (as provided with a Flowtron machine) or by regular bandaging is needed. The latter is more time consuming and requires considerable skill, but is probably more effective in reducing the oedema. After active therapy the arm is placed in an elasticated compression sleeve. This should be measured on an individual basis for each patient. Antibiotics should be prescribed early and for longer than usual in patients with infection in a lymphoedematous arm as tissue perfu-

Table 6.11   Axillary recurrence following clearance, radiotherapy and watch policy (from National Surgical Adjuvant Breast Protocol B-04)

	Mx Cl	Mx XRT	Mx
Number of patients	362	352	365
% axillary relapse	1	3	18
10-year survival	46	48	41

Mx = mastectomy, Cl = axillary node clearance, XRT = radiotherapy

sion is reduced. Infusions and chemotherapy injections should be avoided on the side of surgery as should anaesthetic agents.

Brachial plexopathy

This complication may be due in part to overlap of radiotherapy fields which can result in high doses of radiation being delivered to the brachial plexus. With modern planning techniques, treatment schedules and newer equipment this complication is rare. Brachial plexopathy can also be due to apical axillary recurrence; this complication is much less common if initial treatment of axillary disease has been optimal.

Reduced range of movement

Both surgery and radiotherapy are associated with reduction in the range of movement of the shoulder in some patients and about 5% develop a frozen shoulder. This can be minimized by regular exercise programmes developed and supervised by physiotherapists. Patients with a frozen shoulder require a prolonged course of intensive physiotherapy.

Predicting which patients will have involved axillary nodes

There is a direct relationship between tumour size and the presence of lymph node metastases (Fig. 5.5). It is of interest that tumours detected by screening are less likely to have axillary metastases at each individual size than symptomatic patients. For this reason it has become standard practice in many units for patients with impalpable breast cancer to perform an axillary node sample or a level I dissection, whereas those with palpable disease are treated with a level III clearance. For patients undergoing a mastectomy for invasive breast cancer an axillary clearance is indicated, thus reducing the need for post-operative radiotherapy in the majority. This is particularly important when immediate breast reconstruction is being performed as radiotherapy will significantly affect the final cosmetic result. This goes someway to meeting the aims of limiting the morbidity of surgery and/or radiotherapy to those who require it. It is evident that if patients are node negative then it would be best to identify this group by the most limited surgery, such as an axillary node sample, whereas in patients who are node positive it would be ideal for them to have an axillary node clearance as this would both stage and treat the axilla. What is required are pre-operative assessments which will allow those patients with axillary node disease to be identified. At present no such investigations are available.

Techniques of axillary surgery

Sentinel node biopsy. Injection of radiolabelled (technetium) sulphur colloid and/or a blue dye into the tumour or the skin overlying it, allows identification of the sentinel node either by intraoperative visual inspection or radiation monitoring using a gamma detecting probe. For patients with breast cancer, one or two nodes are usually identified. Use of either modality alone reduces the sensitivity of the examination. This procedure involves a small axillary incision and can be performed under local anaesthesia although usually follows resection of the primary breast cancer. It would appear that the technique will benefit patients with small tumours (under 2 cm) where there is a lower likelihood of axillary involvement, thus sparing them a formal axillary clearance if the sentinel node(s) is clear.

Axillary node sampling. This is usually performed through a separate axillary incision in the skin crease of the axilla and should ideally be undertaken immediately prior to the wide local excision. The axilla is entered and the tail of the breast and lower axilla palpated. If nodes cannot be identified easily, the edges of pectoralis major and latissimus dorsi muscles should be formally identified and a finger passed round behind the lower axillary fat, which is situated between these two muscles; this makes nodes in this fat easier to feel. Starting from the lower axilla at least four palpable nodes are excised and sent separately for histology. If four nodes are not palpable in the lower axilla (level I) then palpable nodes from higher in the axilla (level II, level III or the interpectoral region, see Fig. 1.5) are excised. It is important to appreciate that an axillary node sample is not merely a level I dissection but samples palpable nodes from any level of the axilla. This should allow detection of the few patients who have level II or III involvement but uninvolved level I axillary nodes — the so-called skip metastases. Haemostasis in the axilla is secured with diathermy. No drains are necessary and the wound is closed in layers with absorbable sutures.

Axillary node clearance. Prior to the start of the operation the arm is draped so it can be moved during the procedure. As with axillary node sampling, axillary node clearance is usually performed through a separate incision, before the wide local excision. A lazy S incision is made along the skin creases of the axilla. The skin incision is deepened and skin flaps dissected to the edges of the pectoralis major and latissimus dorsi muscles. The pectoralis minor muscle is cleared of tissue. This is best performed with the arm placed above the patient's head, with retraction on the pectoralis major muscle if the pectoralis minor muscle is not to be divided. If there is evidence of extensive nodal disease, division of pectoralis minor on the coracoid process allows a more thorough clearance to be performed. The front of the axillary vein is identified and the contents of the axilla below the vein are cleared to the apex of the axilla preserving the long thoracic nerve, the thoracodorsal nerve and vessels and, if possible, the intercostobrachial nerve. A combination of blunt and sharp dissection, with division of structures between ligaclips, allows a speedy and effective clearance of the axilla. The undersurface of the pectoralis major muscle should be carefully palpated and any palpable interpectoral nodes excised. Dissection of the lower axillary contents should continue into the axillary tail of the breast. A single suction drain is placed in the axilla and remains *in situ* until the volume of fluid in the drain is less than 50 ml in 24 h. The wound is closed with absorbable sutures.

Recommended management of axillary nodes in patients with operable invasive breast cancer is outlined in Table 6.12.

Treatment of internal mammary and supraclavicular nodes

The value of prophylactic irradiation of the internal mammary and supraclavicular nodes is unproven. For anatomical and geometric

Table 6.12 Recommended management of axillary nodes in patients with operable breast cancer

---

Premenopausal women
Axillary staging
- Mandatory for all patients

Level II dissection
- Patients with palpable, clinically involved nodes
- Patients undergoing mastectomy and reconstruction

Choice of level III dissection, axillary sampling or sentinel node biopsy
- All other patients

Postmenopausal women
Level III dissection
- Patients with palpable, clinically involved nodes

Choice of level III dissection, axillary sampling or sentinel node biopsy
- All other patients with palpable breast cancers

Choice of axillary sampling, sentinel node biopsy or watch policy
- Patients with impalpable cancers (<1 cm in diameter)

---

reasons, the supraclavicular nodes can readily be included when axillary radiotherapy is given and, providing there is no overlap of
fields, has little in the way of morbidity. Such treatment reduces the
rate of supraclavicular recurrence but has no impact on survival.
Over 90% of women with metastases in the internal mammary nodes
have axillary node involvement. Of the 5–10% who have internal
mammary node involvement in isolation, most have tumours involving the medial half of the breast. The internal mammary nodes can
be irradiated only by means of complex fields that include the heart
and these nodes are therefore no longer covered routinely in
radiotherapy fields after mastectomy or wide local excision.

ADJUVANT THERAPY AND OPERABLE BREAST CANCER

In those with operable breast cancer, systemic treatment can be
given following surgery and/or radiotherapy — adjuvant treatment,
or in patients with large operable breast cancers, therapy can be
given initially (**primary medical therapy** or **neoadjuvant therapy**)
prior to locoregional therapy. Where the effectiveness of adjuvant
therapy has been demonstrated in clinical trials, the benefits of primary systemic therapy are still under evaluation.

Primary medical therapy

One potential problem with primary systemic therapy is that, if the
diagnosis of cancer is made by FNAC alone, *in situ* disease could be
overtreated. A biopsy to obtain a histological diagnosis of invasive
cancer should therefore be obtained before embarking on primary
medical treatment. There is no evidence that leaving a primary
tumour in the breast during primary systemic treatment increases a
patient's anxiety. The advantages and disadvantages of adjuvant and
primary systemic treatments are outlined in Table 6.13.

Primary systemic therapy was introduced initially as treatment
for inoperable and locally advanced disease to achieve tumour
reduction and to make locally advanced tumours operable. Its use
has now been extended to patients with large operable breast cancers in an attempt to avoid mastectomy. Response rates ranging
from 62% in tumours larger than 5 cm to 93% in tumours from 3–4
cm have been reported. After chemotherapy, breast-conserving
surgery (quadrantectomy) was possible in 91% of patients in one
series with just over 73% of patients with tumours over 5 cm becoming candidates for breast conservation. At 18 months, only one out
of 201 patients treated by primary systemic therapy, quadrantect-

Table 6.13   Advantages and disadvantages of adjuvant and primary systemic treatment

Systemic treatment	Advantages	Disadvantages
Adjuvant	Proven efficiency	Uncertainty whether treatment is effective in individual patients
	Prognostic information available after surgery	
Primary	Allows direct assessment of effectiveness	Loss of prognostic information
		May overtreat *in situ* disease (if diagnosis made by FNAC alone)
	Tumour shrinkage may allow breast conservation	

omy and post-operative radiotherapy suffered a local recurrence. Response during treatment is assessed according to the criteria of the International Union Against Cancer (UICC) (Table 6.14). Both the primary tumour and lymph node metastases can be shown to respond and invasive cancers seem to be more sensitive to chemotherapy than *in situ* disease.

Chemotherapy

Regimens for primary systemic therapy generally have been the same as those used for adjuvant treatment with about 50% of patients showing a partial response, 20–30% a complete clinical response and a small number (about 10–15%) achieving a complete pathological response. There is preliminary evidence that continuous infusional chemotherapy with agents, such as fluorouracil, com-

Table 6.14   World Health Organisation's definition of objective response

- Complete clinical response
  Disappearance of palpable disease

- Partial response
  Decrease of ≥50% in total size of tumour

- No change
  Decrease of <50% or increase of <25% in total size of tumour at 6 months

- Progressive disease
  Increase of ≥25% in total size of palpable lesion

bined with intermittent agents, such as epirubicin and cisplatin, achieve even higher response rates (over 90%) when compared with standard regimens of bolus chemotherapy. This is a more complicated regimen requiring insertion of a central venous line (or peripherally inserted central catheter [PICC]) and inpatient delivery of the platinum containing compound.

Primary hormonal therapy

Tamoxifen (20 mg a day by mouth) produces a partial response in 75% of elderly patients with ER-positive tumours and a complete clinical response in 15%. Current studies are evaluating primary therapy with the new aromatase inhibitors (anastrozole, letrozole or vorozole). Preliminary evidence suggests that these agents are at least as effective as tamoxifen. The use of luteinizing hormone releasing hormone (LHRH) agonists as primary medical treatment for premenopausal women with ER-positive tumours is also under evaluation. Few patients show a complete pathological response after hormonal therapy but the side-effects are generally much less than with chemotherapy.

Outcome

Tumours will show either a useful response or progression within 12 weeks of primary medical treatment. To ensure that women with progressive disease are detected as early as possible, clinical and ultrasonographic assessment of tumour volume should be performed at monthly intervals. At present, there is no evidence that primary systemic therapy produces any survival advantage and, unless in trials, its use should be restricted to large, operable breast cancers or locally advanced breast cancer.

HORMONAL THERAPY

Introduction

Oestrogen and progesterone regulate the growth and differentiation of normal breast tissue. Evidence for this includes a reduced breast cancer risk in women who have an early menopause and an increased risk of breast cancer in women treated with oestrogen replacement therapy. Oestrogens play an important role in the progression of breast cancer and exert their effect on cells through binding to specific nuclear receptors. Oestrogen receptors and, to a lesser extent, progesterone receptors determine the response to endocrine therapy, given either as treatment for locally advanced or metastatic breast cancer or given as an adjuvant after locoregional therapy. Patients with oestrogen-receptor positive tumours have between a 50% and 70% chance of responding to hormonal therapy and this increases to over 70% in patients whose tumours have both oestrogen and progesterone receptors.

The major source of oestrogens in premenopausal women is the ovary. Levels of oestrogen in postmenopausal women are much lower and oestrogens are synthesized peripherally, principally in fat (including breast fat), skin, muscle and liver from androstenedione which is produced in the adrenal gland. The production of oestrogens requires the presence of the hormone aromatase.

Historical background

Hormonal therapy, or perhaps more correctly anti-hormonal therapy, for breast cancer dates back to 1896 when Beatson treated six premenopausal women with metastatic breast cancer by oophorectomy and documented regression of skin nodules in two. Oophorectomy is not effective in postmenopausal women and adrenalectomy was formerly used in these patients as a means of interrupting hormone synthesis.

Current hormonal therapies and agents

Oophorectomy

This procedure can be performed surgically, medically or with radiotherapy. It increases survival from breast cancer in the adjuvant setting but is now rarely used in advanced disease where it has been superseded by LHRH agonists. LHRH agonists suppress ovarian production by desensitizing pituitary LHRH receptors. Administration of these agents stimulates gonadotrophin production initially but thereafter blocks release of FSH and LH with a net decrease in production of both oestrogen and progesterone from the ovary resulting in endocrine blockade with cessation of menstruation. These drugs only have activity in premenopausal women. The advantage of surgery is that tissue is obtained which can be examined histologically for metastases. If laproscopy is used then extensive visualization of the abdominal cavity is possible.

Tamoxifen

Tamoxifen is a synthetic partial oestrogen agonist which acts primarily by binding to the oestrogen receptor. It is the most widely used hormonal treatment for breast cancer. It has a half-life of 7 days and it takes approximately 4 weeks for the drug to reach a steady state in the plasma. The standard dose is 20 mg once a day, although at this dose there are wide variations in plasma concentrations of the drug between individual patients. Between 0% and 10% of patients with ER-negative tumours apparently have a response to this drug. Technical problems associated with ER assays and lack of quality control may account for some of the variations of reported response rates. Response rates with tamoxifen are similar to other endocrine agents but some tumours develop resistance to tamoxifen. Tumours which have become resistant to tamoxifen do not appear to lose their ER and overgrowth of ER-negative clones can only explain the development of tamoxifen resistance.

Although tamoxifen appears to be antagonistic in its action on breast cancer cells, it has oestrogen agonist activity at other sites which accounts for both the benefits and side-effects of the treatment. Benefits include preservation of bone density, decrease in plasma cholesterol levels and an associated reduction in cardiovascular morbidity (both agonist effects) as well as a 35–40% decrease in second primary breast cancers (antagonistic effect). Only 3% of patients given tamoxifen stop taking the drug because of side-effects.

Hot flushes are among the most common complaints of treatment. Megestrol acetate 20 mg twice a day appears to be effective at reducing this troublesome symptom. In premenopausal women, tamoxifen can decrease vaginal secretions and produce atrophy and vaginal dryness. This should be treated initially with a non-hormonal cream (such as Replens) but if this is not effective and symptoms are severe, pessaries containing oestrogen should be prescribed. Systemic absorption of oestrogens is of potential concern but appears minimal with Vagifem. Tamoxifen has oestrogenic effects on the uterus which accounts for the approximately fourfold increase in the risk of uterine cancer in women on this drug. The number of endometrial cancers developing on tamoxifen is less than the number of contralateral breast cancers tamoxifen prevents (Table 6.15). In the USA, women have endometrial screening prior to starting tamoxifen but this is not common practice in the UK and Europe. There is in fact no evidence that this screening is necessary. Although placebo-controlled trials have not shown an excessive weight gain in women on tamoxifen, this is the most common complaint of women on long-term treatment.

Table 6.15   Direct estimates of reduction in the annual odds of recurrence and death among women aged less than 50 in trials of adjuvant therapy (from EBCTGC overview)

Adjuvant therapy	Reductions % (SD) in annual odds of		
	No. aged <50 years	Recurrence or prior death	Death from any cause
Trials of single modality therapy with untreated controls			
• Polychemotherapy vs nil	2976	37 (5)	27 (6)
• Ovarian suppression vs nil	878	30 (9)	28 (9)
• Tamoxifen (mean 2.6 years) vs nil	2216	27 (7)	17 (10)
All tamoxifen trials, including those in which both arms also received chemotherapy			
• Tamoxifen 1 year	2478	5 (7)	4 (8)
• Tamoxifen 2 years	4794	10 (5)	4 (6)
• Tamoxifen >2 years	1311	43 (11)	27 (17)

Retinal problems have occasionally been reported but are rare. Tamoxifen appears to cause liver cancer in rats but this is apparently not a problem in humans.

Tamoxifen has been used both as an adjuvant and as therapy for metastatic breast cancer in premenopausal women. Tamoxifen does not appear to have a major effect on FSH and LH levels but oestradiol and oestrone levels are increased. Many premenopausal women taking tamoxifen still have regular menses and it is important to advise that pregnancy can occur. In the treatment of metastatic disease, tamoxifen produces equivalent rates of response to oophorectomy and, in the adjuvant setting, it appears to improve survival of premenopausal women, who have hormone receptor-positive tumours with little apparent benefit in ER-negative tumours.

Other synthetic anti-oestrogens have been developed and some such as toremifene are in clinical use. Other non-steroidal anti-oestrogens including draloxifene, raloxifene and idoxifene are in clinical trials. Some of the newer agents retain agonist effects on bone but have little effect on the uterus. Pure anti-oestrogens have been developed, such as ICI 182170 (Faslodex); early clinical trials have shown it to be well tolerated and effective.

Aromatase inhibitors

The production of oestrogen requires the presence and activity of the aromatase enzyme. Oestrogen production in postmenopausal women is by peripheral aromatization of androgens produced from the adrenal gland. A number of aromatase inhibitors have been used in the treatment of breast cancer and a number are under development.

Aminoglutethimide was the first aromatase inhibitor to be used. This is not, however, a pure aromatase inhibitor and also blocks production of cortisol. It is used less commonly now because of side-effects. The second agent to be used clinically was 4-hydroxy-androstenedione (Formestane). This is 30–60 times more potent than aminoglutethimide at inhibiting aromatase, but studies showed that this drug inhibits circulating oestradiol levels by 60%. The problem with 4-hydroxyandrostenedione is that is has to be given by intramuscular injection at a dose of 250 mg twice weekly.

Newer aromatase inhibitors

The third generation aromatase inhibitors include the non-steroidal inhibitors with imidazole or triazole structures. These agents have better specificity for the aromatase enzyme and are much less toxic than aminoglutethimide. The agents currently licensed include anastrozole and letrozole which produce between 96.7% and 98.9% aromatase inhibition. Vorozole is another agent which is currently in trials but appears to be at least as effective as anastrozole and letrozole. A new steroidal aromatase inhibitor, exemestane, is currently also in clinical trials.

Aromatase inhibitors have been shown to be effective in treating breast cancer that has ceased to respond to tamoxifen with a survival advantage over progestogens which are the current second line hormonal agents.

Progestogens

These agents are used in the treatment of metastatic breast cancer. Medroxyprogesterone acetate (MPA) and megestrol acetate are the best known agents. Response rates are similar to that of tamoxifen, when used as a second line agent. The mechanisms of action of progestogens are unknown but they may:

- Interfere with the binding of oestrogen to the oestrogen receptor.
- Accelerate oestrogen catabolism.
- Interfere with aromatization of androgens to oestrogens.

The reason these agents are reserved for second or third-line treatment is the frequency with which they cause side-effects. The major side-effect of megestrol acetate is weight gain, but vaginal spotting can also be a problem. The standard dose of megestrol acetate is 160 mg once a day. Anti-progestogens are currently in clinical trials.

CHEMOTHERAPY AGENTS

Many active agents are available for the treatment of breast cancer and numerous combination chemotherapy regimes have been reported. Certain drugs form the cornerstone of treatment and include the following:

Anthracyclines

Doxorubicin

Anthracyclines have long been considered to be the most active single agents in the treatment of breast cancer. The anti-tumour antibiotic, doxorubicin (adriamycin), is the most widely used of these agents. Side-effects include myelosuppression and mucositis. Although it is usually given as a bolus once every 3 weeks, weekly administration allows some intensification of dosage and possibly reduces cardiac toxicity. Doxorubicin produces alopecia in most patients.

Epirubicin

This is a semi-synthetic doxorubicin stereo-isomer. Its single agent response rate is comparable to that of doxorubicin. It is associated with less cardiac toxicity and is used most frequently in combination regimens such as ECF (epirubicin, cisplatin, 5-fluorouracil).

Mitoxantrone

The cumulative dose and dose rate of doxorubicin are limited by cardiac toxicity and so other anthracycline analogues have been developed to circumvent this problem. Although mitoxantrone is reported to produce less cardiac toxicity than doxorubicin, clinical trials have demonstrated cardiac effects with increasing doses. Side-effects are similar but less common than those with doxorubicin. Mitoxantrone is often used in combination with mitomycin-C and methotrexate (MMM).

Cyclophosphamide

Cyclophosphamide is inert until activated by microsomal enzymes in the liver which then produce the potent alkylating cytotoxic metabolite, phosphoramide mustard. Although cyclophosphamide is an active single agent, it is usually used in combination regimes such as CMF (cyclophosphamide, 5-fluorouracil and methotrexate). Specific side-effects include mucositis and occasionally chemical cystitis.

5-Fluorouracil (5-FU)

This is a pyrimidine analogue which has been used in cancer chemotherapy for more than 30 years. The drug first has to be metabolized and then binds to an enzyme — thymidine synthatase — thus inhibiting DNA synthesis. In early trials, 5-FU was administered as a bolus but more recently it has been used as an infusional therapy, initially over 24 h, then over 5 days and now continuously for many months. Specific problems with continuous 5-FU include the hand foot syndrome where the patient develops erythema and eventually blistering of the epithelium over the hands and feet, and mucositis. It is the only drug currently available that can be infused continuously for long periods.

Methotrexate

Methotrexate is an analogue of folic acid and works by indirectly blocking thymidylate synthesis. In breast cancer it is used primarily in the CMF and MMM regimes.

Platinum compounds

Platinum compounds were first used in the treatment of germ cell tumours. These compounds work by forming adducts with DNA which inhibit replication. Toxicity is a problem with the platinum compounds and includes peripheral neuropathy, renal toxicity and ototoxicity. Carboplatin is reported to have similar efficacy to cisplatin but fewer toxic effects. It is most frequently used in the ECF regimen.

Mitomycin

Mitomycin is an anti-tumour antibiotic. Its main problem is cumulative mylotoxicity.

Taxoids

Paclitaxel (Taxol) is a novel chemotherapeutic agent derived from the Pacific yew tree. It has a unique mechanism of action and stabilizes microtubular assembly which prevents cell division. Another semi-synthetic taxoid, docetaxol (Taxotere) has been derived from the European yew tree. Dose-limiting toxicity seems to be myelo-suppression. These agents are very active against breast cancer although to date the interest in their activity has been based on observations in anthracycline-resistant or refractory patients. Continued trials will define their role and the correct dosing schedule in primary and adjuvant combination therapy. They are currently very expensive.

Complications of chemotherapy

The complications and side-effects include alopecia, neutropaenia, nausea and vomiting. There are also specific side-effects for each agent which are not discussed here.

Alopecia

This can be expected with higher doses of cyclophosphamide and mitozantrone and at most commonly used doses of doxorubicin (adriamycin). This may be reduced by scalp cooling using either cold packs or, preferably, a purpose-built, scalp-cooling machine.

Neutropaenia

This is to be expected and regular blood counts should be obtained. The nadir (lowest point) for most regimens is known and patients may need prophylactic antibiotics to cover this period. Dose reductions and delays may be necessary if the white cell count falls below defined limits. The death of a patient through uncontrolled infection due to neutropaenia offsets any benefit in reduction of mortality for the population being treated.

The use of haematological growth factors prepared by genetic engineering techniques can shorten the time a patient is neutropaenic and reduce the need for antibiotics and hospital stays. Granulocyte colony stimulating factor (G-CSF) is more commonly used than GMCSF (macrophages included) but the exact role of these growth factors is currently being evaluated.

Nausea and vomiting

These are among the more unpleasant side-effects of chemotherapy. The percentage of patients experiencing nausea differs with the different combinations of chemotherapy and some regimens require few or no antiemetic measures. Others, such as cisplatin and high-dose doxorubicin are highly emetogenic. Recognized antiemetic regimens are shown in Table 6.16. The arrival of the 5-HT$_3$ receptor antagonists has reduced the problem to manageable levels. It seems reasonable to reserve these agents for highly emetogenic regimens and for those whose nausea cannot be controlled by more conventional measures such as sea-bands (which use stimulation of the PS acupuncture point on the volar aspect of the wrist), regular metoclopramide, benzodiazapines, dexamethasone and cannabis derivatives.

Younger women are more at risk of nausea and vomiting. The aim of treatment is to prevent them ever experiencing it so as to avoid the condition of anticipatory nausea and vomiting which can be particularly upsetting.

ADJUVANT SYSTEMIC TREATMENT

This is aimed at the second fundamental part of breast cancer treatment (attempting to reduce the systemic load) and requires the administration of an intervention (chemotherapy, endocrine therapy or endocrine ablation) to an otherwise well patient. These treat-

Table 6.16   Antiemetic regimens for chemotherapy-induced nausea and vomiting

Regimen	Administration
Low emetogenic regimes (low-dose epirubicin)	Oral metoclopramide (if necessary)
Moderately emetogenic (CMF, MMM doxorubicin, high-dose epirubicin)	Dexamethasone 8–16 mg intravenously before or after chemotherapy and metoclopramide* followed by oral dexamethasone (4 mg t.d.s. for 3 days) and metoclopramide (10 mg t.d.s. for 3 days) to take at home. Metoclopramide may be continued if necessary. Or ondansetron 8 mg intravenously or granisetron 3 mg intravenously before chemotherapy with dexamethasone intravenously and followed by oral dexamethasone
Highly emetogenic regimens (not often used in routine management of breast cancer other than some centres using cisplatin regimens but used for high-dose doxorubicin and patients who fail on the above regimens)	Ondansetron 8 mg intravenously or granisetron 3 mg intravenously before chemotherapy with dexamethasone intravenously and followed by oral dexamethasone

*low dose 20–30 mg intravenously or high dose 100 mg infusion — may need to give 1 mg benztropine intravenously in younger patients receiving high dose to combat extrapyramidal side-effects

ments all have potential side-effects and a risk-benefit analysis needs to be made on the patient's behalf.

The translation of benefits for such treatments from large trials which have shown improvements in overall survival and time to relapse to an individual, can be difficult for both patient and clinician. A node-positive woman who relapses at, for example, 36 months despite receiving adjuvant chemotherapy may not feel that 6 months of chemotherapy was worthwhile even if, statistically, she would otherwise have relapsed at 24 months.

The role of chemotherapy and endocrine therapy is now reasonably well established and newer agents are being studied.

Adjuvant systemic therapy for operable breast cancer

The effect of adjuvant therapy has been shown in clinical trials but its effect in individuals cannot be assessed as there is no overt disease to monitor. Because small randomized trials can produce misleading results, data from all trials have been analysed in an overview and meta-analysis. Large numbers of patients included in such an analysis provide great statistical power enabling this analysis to detect modest advantage of one treatment over another.

Adjuvant endocrine therapy and chemotherapy in women with operable breast cancer each reduce the annual risks of death by about 30% for at least 10 years. Benefits of adjuvant therapy may add up to 10 extra women alive at 10 years for every woman with stage II disease and five extra women alive at 10 years for every 100 women with stage I disease.

The relative reductions of mortality are the same in axillary node-negative and positive women. This suggests that adjuvant therapy is equally active in both high- and low-risk groups. Absolute reduction in death rate depends on the chance of a woman dying from the disease. A 30% reduction in the relative risk of odds of dying reduces a 10% mortality at 10 years by 3% and a 60% mortality at 10 years by 20%. The shape of disease free and overall survival curves over time indicates that for most patients the benefit is that of a delay in the onset of recurrence rather than long-term cure.

Adjuvant hormone therapy

Results from the Early Breast Cancer Trialists' Overview demonstrate that, in women under 50 years of age, ovarian suppression as the sole adjuvant therapy is associated with a 30% reduction in the annual risk of death, this effect lasting for at least 15 years. The

Overview suggests that prolonged tamoxifen therapy appears to produce benefits in premenopausal women as well as post-menopausal women but of a lesser order. Benefits of oophorectomy appear greatest in ER-positive patients. The evidence that is available on duration of tamoxifen suggests that it should be used for 5 years.

Postmenopausal patients

Compared to a 6% reduction in annual risk of death in women below the age of 50, tamoxifen produces a 20% reduction in annual odds of death in women aged 50 or older. The optimum duration of tamoxifen in this group is 5 years. There appears to be a significant interaction between the ER status of the tumour and the benefit obtained from tamoxifen in postmenopausal patients. Although patients with ER-poor tumours may obtain a small benefit.

Chemotherapy

The Overview concluded that when using chemotherapy, a combination of drugs produced better results than a single drug alone and that six courses produces similar benefits to more prolonged treatment schedules. Pre-operative chemotherapy has not yet been shown to produce a survival benefit.

Premenopausal patients

Adjuvant chemotherapy appears to produce similar benefits in odds reductions of death as oophorectomy (Table 6.15). Data from a Scottish trial suggest that the greatest benefit from chemotherapy is in patients with ER-negative tumours. Adjuvant chemotherapy given for at least 2 months produces a highly significant 36% reduction in annual odds of recurrence in women aged under 50 and a 24% reduction in the annual odds of death. Chemotherapy appears to be most effective in younger patients. One-third or more of recurrence and one-quarter of all of the deaths in premenopausal women appear to be avoided or delayed at 10 years by adjuvant chemotherapy.

Postmenopausal patients

Ten-year survival data do show a statistically significant reduction in recurrence and improved survival in postmenopausal patients given adjuvant chemotherapy. The benefits are however less than in premenopausal women and are less pronounced as the age of the patient increases. Too few women aged over 70 years of age were included in the Overview to provide a valid estimate of the effects of adjuvant chemotherapy in these patients.

Optimal regimen for adjuvant chemotherapy

The most commonly used treatment is six cycles of CMF over 6 months. Studies have demonstrated that four cycles of adjuvant chemotherapy appear to be as effective as six cycles of CMF. Interestingly, in this direct comparison the days of nausea were fewer with the CMF regimen; cardiac toxicity was not a major problem although alopecia was worse with the adjuvant chemotherapy regimen.

In a randomized trial from Milan of patients with four or more positive nodes, two sequences of doxorubicin and CMF were compared; the sequences were doxorubicin for four cycles followed by intravenous CMF for eight courses or CMF for two cycles followed by doxorubicin for one cycle repeated to a total of 12 courses. This study demonstrated a highly significant improvement in disease free and overall survival in the patients treated initially with four courses of doxorubicin. The survival curve of the patients having a sequential regimen actually flattened out a few years after the start of treatment suggesting that this regimen may be curing some patients. Although no CMF arm alone was included in this trial, comparison with early results suggests that the sequence of doxorubicin followed by CMF is a potent regimen for high-risk, node-positive patients.

Dose-intensive adjuvant chemotherapy

In 1981 the Milan group reported that only those patients who received at least 85% of their planned CMF dose benefited significantly from adjuvant chemotherapy, whereas those receiving less than 65% of the planned dose had the same disease free and overall survival as the control group treated by surgery alone. Later in the retrospective analysis of published randomized trials, Hryniuk and Levine showed a direct correlation between survival and dose intensity. Dose intensity has been investigated in a variety of studies and one of these patients received three different doses of CMF. After a median follow up of 3.4 years, the higher and moderate dose-intensity regimes yielded superior disease free and overall survivals when compared with the low dose; the low-dose chemotherapy however was well below the intensity which most oncologists would have considered acceptable. It may be therefore that there is a threshold rather than a dose-response effect, i.e. there is a minimum dose below which cytotoxics are not effective.

Studies of dose intensity using extremely high-dose chemotherapy and autologous bone marrow transplant or peripheral stem cell rescue are being evaluated. A non-randomized study from Duke University estimated a 72% 3-year disease free survival with high-dose chemotherapy and marrow rescue. Although this was superior to the survival of local historical controls, the efficacy of this treatment remains unproven and it should be restricted to patients entering randomized clinical trials.

Current view on endocrine therapy

The benefit of adjuvant therapy in any individual patient and possible treatment side-effects, long term toxicities and their impact on quality of life, need to be taken into consideration when selecting adjuvant therapy for individual patients. The current philosophy is to stratify patients in relation to their risk of recurrence and death, and to tailor the adjuvant treatment to that risk. Patients can be stratified on the basis of number of involved nodes (Table 6.17) using tumour size and grade to stratify the node-negative group. Alternatively, patients can be stratified on the basis of a single index such as the Nottingham Prognostic Index which combines tumour size, histological tumour grade and node status. Having identified different risk groups, adjuvant therapy is then tailored to that risk. An outline of the current recommendations for adjuvant treatment for patients with operable breast cancer is given in Table 6.18.

Table 6.17   Definitions of risk groups and associated risk of relapse

Risk group	Definition	Survival without relapse after 5 years
Node-negative patients		
● Low risk	Tumour <1 cm in diameter	>90%
● Intermediate risk	Tumour >1 cm, grade I or II	75–80%
● High risk	Tumour >1 cm, grade III	0–60%
Node-positive patients		
● Low and intermediate risk	1–3 axillary nodes involved	40–50%
● High risk	4–9 axillary nodes involved	20–30%
● Very high risk	>10 axillary nodes involved	10–15%

Table 6.18 Adjuvant treatment for patients with breast cancer

Risk group	Premenopausal patients	Postmenopausal patients
Node-negative patients		
● Low risk	Tamoxifen or no treatment	Tamoxifen or no treatment
● Intermediate risk	Tamoxifen	Tamoxifen
● High risk	Chemotherapy★ (with or without tamoxifen) *or* Ovarian ablation (with or without tamoxifen) if tumour is ER-positive	Tamoxifen (with or without chemotherapy)
Node-positive patients		
● Low and intermediate risk	Chemotherapy★ (with or without tamoxifen) *or* Ovarian ablation (with or without tamoxifen) if tumour is ER-positive *or* Chemotherapy★ and ovarian ablation (with or without tamoxifen)	Tamoxifen with or without chemotherapy
● High and very high risk	Consider more intensive chemotherapy† (with or without tamoxifen)	Tamoxifen and chemotherapy if fit

★For example, cyclophosphamide, methotrexate and fluorouracil
†For example, regimen containing anthracycline. Some units are investigating use of intensive chemotherapy supported by rescue of bone marrow or peripheral stem cells for patients at very high risk

TREATMENT OF ELDERLY PATIENTS

About 40% of all breast cancers occur in women over the age of 70. The cancers that develop in older women are as aggressive as those in younger patients. Traditionally these patients were treated by tamoxifen alone but long-term local control at 5 years is less than 30% and this is no longer satisfactory. The average life expectancy of a 70-year-old woman is 14.5 years and that of an 80-year-old woman is 8.5 years. Elderly women with breast cancer therefore should be treated in a similar way to younger patients. Few patients are truly unfit for surgery because wide local excision and even mastectomy can be performed under local or regional anaesthesia with sedation. There is no evidence to suggest that elderly patients do not tolerate radiotherapy as well as younger patients and when radiotherapy is given it should be given in a radical dose.

As elderly patients often have ER-positive breast cancers, many of the patients who present with large breast cancers can be treated by primary systemic (neoadjuvant) endocrine therapy, for an initial period of 3 months and this then allows less extensive surgery to be performed. Although this approach does not appear to improve survival, it does limit the morbidity of treatment. If the patient is to have a mastectomy, this should be combined in most instances with a level III axillary clearance as this has a similar post-operative morbidity (less than 1%) to simple mastectomy and is associated with a significantly lower rate of local recurrence. The standard therapy in adjuvant patients has been tamoxifen alone. It is clear, however, that some of these elderly patients are very fit and, if they are considered to be at high risk of systemic recurrence, then it seems inappropriate to deny them potentially beneficial chemotherapy.

A summary of the management of elderly patients with breast cancer is presented in Table 6.19.

Table 6.19   Management of elderly patients with breast cancer

Tumour stage and size	Treatment options
T_1 or $T_2 \leq 4$ cm size, N_{0-1}, M_0	Wide local excision, node sampling or clearance, and radiotherapy *or* Mastectomy, node clearance and adjuvant tamoxifen
$T_2 > 4$ cm or T_3, N_{0-1}, M_0: *Oestrogen receptor:*	
• Positive	Mastectomy, node clearance and adjuvant tamoxifen *or* Tamoxifen and then, if tumour regresses, wide local excision, node sampling or clearance and radiotherapy
• Unknown, negative or no response to tamoxifen	Mastectomy, node clearance, and adjuvant tamoxifen
T_4, N_2, M_0: *Oestrogen receptor:*	
• Positive	Tamoxifen
• Unknown, negative or no respose to tamoxifen	Radical radiotherapy or *in selected patients* Mastectomy and radiotherapy Possibly chemotherapy
Any T, any N, M_1: *Oestrogen receptor:*	
• Positive or unknown	Tamoxifen and symptomatic treatment
• Negative	Symptomatic treatment and possibly low-dose epirubicin or mitozantrone
Very elderly or infirm patients	Tamoxifen

TREATMENT OF BREAST CANCER DURING PREGNANCY

This occurs at a frequency of between one and three in every 10 000 pregnancies. Twenty-five per cent of all breast cancers in women aged less than 35 are associated with pregnancy in that they develop either during or within 1 year of pregnancy. There is no evidence that breast cancer during pregnancy is more aggressive than breast cancer at other times, but diagnosis is often delayed because of the difficulty of identifying a discrete mass in enlarging breasts. This means that women tend to present with cancers at a later stage and about 65% have involved nodes. Treatment during the first two trimesters is usually a modified radical mastectomy. Radiotherapy should not be delivered during pregnancy. Chemotherapy can be given but is associated with a small risk of foetal damage, particularly in the early stages of pregnancy. Breast cancer in the third trimester can be managed either by immediate surgery or by monitoring the tumour, delivering the baby early at 30–32 weeks and instituting treatment after delivery. This allows patients with large or locally advanced breast cancers to have primary systemic treatment which can sometimes cause regression of the disease to allow less extensive surgery to be performed.

PREGNANCY AFTER TREATMENT OF BREAST CANCER

There is limited information on the effect of pregnancy on the outcome of patients with breast cancer. None of the studies performed so far has demonstrated that pregnancy does have an adverse effect but there are clearly theoretical risks of increasing circulating hormone levels in these patients. It is generally recommended that there should be a delay of 2–3 years between initial treatment for breast cancer and pregnancy because most relapses (80%) occur within the first 2 years. Women who are treated by breast conservation (wide local excision and radiotherapy) usually find difficulty breast feeding after this treatment although there are reports of women who have been able to breast feed and there appear to be no deleterious effects from doing this to the mother or baby.

HRT AFTER TREATMENT FOR BREAST CANCER

HRT is normally stopped during the treatment phase and this, coupled with oestrogen blockade, can give rise to severe climacteric symptoms. Treatment with clonidine is often unsuccessful although Megace 20 mg twice a day helps some. HRT can be reintroduced or started if the patient's quality of life is poor without it and may be combined with tamoxifen thus achieving some of the benefits of both agents.

TREATMENT OF PAGET'S DISEASE

Paget's disease is an eczematoid change of the nipple associated with an underlying breast malignancy and it is present in about 1–2% of patients with breast cancer. In half these patients, it is associated with an underlying mass lesion and 90% of such patients will have an invasive carcinoma. For the patients without a mass lesion, 30% will later be found to have an invasive carcinoma and the remainder have *in situ* disease alone.

Paget's disease may be localized or occupy a large area. The lesion should be differentiated from eczema of the nipple. Eczema affects principally the areola and only spreads on to the nipple as a secondary event. In contrast, Paget's disease primarily affects the nipple and only later spreads on to the areola. The treatment of eczema is 0.5–1% hydrocortisone cream and the patient should be advised to wash their bras in hypoallergenic washing products.

If it is not clear on clinical examination whether the disease is likely to be eczema or Paget's, or if Paget's disease is suspected, mammography should be performed to determine if there is an underlying lesion. Imprint cytology (pressing the eczematous lesion on to a slide) or scrape cytology (scraping some of the lesion on to a slide) can sometimes establish the diagnosis. The most reliable method of obtaining a diagnosis is by incisional biopsy removing an elliptical portion of abnormal skin and sending this for pathological examination.

Care must also be taken to distinguish between Paget's disease and direct spread of the invasive carcinoma to the skin of the nipple. Not only do they have different histological appearances but the treatment and outcome also differ. Paget's disease may occupy a large area of the breast (Fig 6.12).

Management

If a mass lesion is present, the appropriate treatment is mastectomy and axillary node clearance (6% of patients with a mass lesion have involved axillary nodes). When Paget's disease is associated with an underlying central lesion, a wide local excision of the nipple, areola and mid-line mass followed by radiotherapy has been reported in small series to give satisfactory control rates, although the standard treatment is mastectomy and remains mastectomy. If no mass lesion is present, the mastectomy or wide local excision should be combined with an axillary node staging procedure such as axillary node sample as many of these patients will actually have DCIS rather than invasive cancer.

Adjuvant therapy is as for other patients with breast cancer (Table 6.18).

MALE BREAST CANCER

Male breast cancer is over 100 times less common than the female variety and represents only 0.7% of all cancers which occur in men. One male breast cancer is seen for every 200 female breast cancers and thus represents 0.5% of all breast cancers. The peak age incidence is 5–10 years older than that in females. The aetiology, like that of female breast cancer, is unknown but there is an increased incidence in patients with Klinefelter syndrome. Gynaecomastia does not seem to be a risk factor.

Clinical features

The presenting features are identical to those in females, patients presenting with a lump, skin or nipple retraction and occasionally nipple discharge. The only difference between the sexes is that, in the male, breast cancers infiltrate skin and the nipple early due to the smaller breast volume (Fig. 6.13). The histology of male breast cancers is similar to that in the female.

Prognosis

The outlook for male breast cancer is similar to that of the female when compared stage for stage but, as noted, the male tends to present with later stage disease.

Treatment

The preferred treatment is a modified radical mastectomy. Often this has to be followed by radiotherapy because of the narrower margins of excision and the often locally advanced nature of the disease. Although the hormonal milieu is different in males, breast cancer still appears to respond well to hormonal therapy and many tumours in males are ER positive. Tamoxifen is therefore the systemic adjuvant treatment of choice following excisional surgery and/or radiotherapy.

For metastatic breast cancer, the options include castration and chemotherapy.

FOLLOW UP OF BREAST CANCER PATIENTS

Local recurrence after mastectomy is most common in the first 2 years and decreases with time. In contrast, local recurrence after breast conservation occurs at a fixed rate each year. Follow-up schedules should take this difference into account. There are three aims of follow up. Firstly, to detect local recurrence at a stage when it can be treated, secondly to deal with psychological problems and to detect these early, and thirdly, to provide a forum for patients to discuss aspects of their disease, particularly the drugs they are receiving and any side-effects that they are experiencing.

Patients with carcinoma in one breast are at high risk of cancer in the other breast and about 0.6% per year develop this. Follow up should include mammography of the opposite breast, performed every 1–2 years. Treated breasts should also be X-rayed on an annual basis. Mammograms can be difficult to interpret after breast conservation because scarring from surgery can produce a stellate opacity which can be difficult to differentiate from cancer recurrence. Magnetic resonance imaging (MRI) is useful in this situation. A sensible follow-up schedule is 6 monthly for the first 2 years and annually thereafter.

OTHER RARE NEOPLASMS

Lymphomas and sarcomas (malignant phyllodes tumours [cystosarcoma], fibrosarcoma and malignant fibrous histiocytoma, angiosarcoma, leiomyosarcoma, liposarcoma and osteosarcoma) occur in the breast but are rare. Sarcomas may develop in an area of breast or skin following radiotherapy. The diagnosis is often suggested by FNAC. Lymphomas are treated by wide excision, radiotherapy and chemotherapy. Sarcomas are best widely excised by mastectomy and followed by radiotherapy, but there is no evidence that chemotherapy is of benefit.

Rare lesions which when excised recur locally include fibromatosis and nodular fasciitis. These have minimal malignant potential and are treated by wide excision.

7. Advanced disease

INTRODUCTION

Advanced disease is usually subdivided into locally advanced (i.e. locally inoperable) and metastatic. Metastatic breast cancer is incurable, although long-term and worthwhile short-term responses can be achieved by the use of appropriate treatments. It is important that quality of life is addressed in treating patients with advanced disease. Tools for measuring this are available and are used in research but have yet to find a place in the routine management of patients.

LOCALLY ADVANCED DISEASE

Definition

Locally advanced disease of the breast is characterized clinically by features suggesting infiltration of the skin or chest wall by tumour or matted involved axillary nodes (Table 7.1). There are two groups

Table 7.1 Clinical features of locally advanced breast cancer

Skin
- Ulceration
- Satellite nodules
- Dermal infiltration
- Peau d'orange
- Erythema over tumour

Chest wall
Tumour fixation to
- Ribs
- Intercostal muscles
- Serratus anterior

Axillary nodes
- Nodes fixed to one another or to other structures

of patients with advanced disease. There is the 'advanced by neglect' group in which a slowly growing tumour has been ignored and allowed to become locally fixed or ulcerated. The other group is the true advanced disease and presents with fixed axillary nodes (N_2) or local signs such as peau d'orange (literally the skin of the orange) or the changes of an inflammatory carcinoma (Fig. 7.1). Some include large T_3 tumours as advanced disease, which is inappropriate as many of these patients will have no evidence of disease elsewhere and can be adequately treated by mastectomy and radiotherapy. It is worthwhile staging this group of patients with bone and liver scans in addition to a chest X-ray (Table 6.3). If the disease is localized then surgery and/or radiotherapy may be curative.

Inflammatory breast cancers can be included in the second category. They traditionally confer a worse prognosis although the use of high-dose chemotherapy is giving promising results.

Treatment

Current treatments have had some impact on local control but have had little overall impact on survival. Patients with hormone sensitive disease have a much longer survival than those with hormone insensitive disease. Local and regional relapse is a major problem in locally advanced disease and affects approximately half of all patients.

Surgery

Some cancers, principally those with direct skin involvement because of position or neglect, are suitable for primary surgical treatment. Mastectomy is generally not indicated in the presence of features of locally advanced disease, but following treatment with a combination of cytotoxic drugs or initial hormonal treatment and surgery may become feasible some weeks or months later. It may be possible to perform a wide excision although mastectomy is the most commonly performed procedure.

The role of systemic and local treatments

The mainstay of local treatments has been radiotherapy because surgery is associated with high rates of local recurrence. Radiotherapy can produce high rates of local remission in both the breast and axilla but when radiotherapy is used alone, only 30% of patients remain free of loco-regional disease at death. By combining appropriate systemic therapy and radiotherapy, response rates of over 80% have been reported and over two-thirds of patients retain loco-regional control at death. Radiotherapy should be given to those few patients managed initially by surgery or those who have operations after a course of systemic therapy.

Choice of systemic treatment

Systemic therapy should be administered as part of a planned programme of combined systemic and local therapies. Factors affecting the choice of systemic therapy for locally advanced breast cancer are outlined in Table 7.2. Standard chemotherapy such as CMF has a reasonable response rate but appears to have little impact on survival. There are some data to suggest that infusional therapies based on 5-fluorouracil (5-FU) combined with doxorubicin with the addition of cyclophosphamide (ACF) or 5-FU combined with epirubicin and cisplatin (ECF) do produce higher local response rates than the intermittent regimes used for adjuvant chemotherapy. Work is currently underway to determine whether intensifying the drug dosage is worthwhile in this group of women and produces an improvement in operability rates, local control and survival.

Primary hormonal therapy can be given to patients with locally advanced breast cancer providing that their cancers are ER positive and appear to be relatively slow growing or indolent. The choice of treatments in these patients is outlined in Table 7.2.

Despite best efforts with combined treatments, a substantial proportion of patients who present with locally advanced disease do develop uncontrolled disease of the chest wall. Impressive local control rates with low toxicity have been reported by giving chemotherapy intra-arterially via the internal mammary or lateral thoracic artery. The drug is administered following radiological placement of a catheter into the vessel which provides the major blood supply

Table 7.2 Factors affecting choice of systemic treatment for locally advanced breast cancer

Hormonal treatment
- Slow growing or indolent disease
- ER-positive cancer
- Elderly or unfit patients

Chemotherapy
- Inflammatory cancer
- ER-negative cancer
- Rapidly progressive cancer

to the tumour. Drugs and doses used are similar to those given intravenously.

LOCALLY RECURRENT DISEASE

The treatment of local recurrences after conservation surgery is discussed on page 130. Recurrence after mastectomy usually occurs in the skin flaps adjacent to the scar and is presumed to arise from viable cells shed at the time of surgery. If radiotherapy was not given at the time of mastectomy it can be used after excision of the recurrence. If the recurrence is small and occurs many years after the original surgery, excision alone may provide control. If the recurrence is in a previously irradiated field, more extensive surgery should be entertained as further radiotherapy will often not be possible (Table 7.3). Standard chemotherapy in this situation is disappointing presumably because the blood supply is diminished although the intra-arterial route may give higher concentrations. 5-FU infused continuously into a central vein via a Hickman line appears to be effective in local recurrence which has proved resistant to more standard treatments. Radical surgery may require resection of underlying structures and reconstruction with flaps. Failure to achieve local control may lead to cancer-en-cuirass where the chest wall is encircled by tumour — a most unpleasant situation for the patient as the tumour often smells or bleeds. Local recurrence can be quite indolent, growing slowly without obvious metastasis elsewhere.

Recurrence in the axilla (usually termed loco-regional relapse) can be treated by surgical clearance if this has not been performed, but is associated with the risk of post-operative lymphoedema. If

Table 7.3   Treatment of local recurrence in chest wall

Type of recurrence	Treatment
Single spot	Excise and consider radiotherapy
Multiple spot	Radiotherapy unless already given or more radical excision (possibly with coverage with myocutaneous flap)
Widespread	Consider radiotherapy unless already given or disease too widespread Appropriate systemic treatment (local application of chemotherapy such as miltefosine applied daily)

the nodes are fixed it may be impossible to operate safely and radiotherapy may be more appropriate if it has not already been given.

Recurrence in the supraclavicular nodes represents dissemination but can often be controlled by radiotherapy. Local surgery has little to contribute in this situation except in making the diagnosis which may be more expeditiously achieved by needle cytology.

Systemic therapy has a role in the treatment of local relapse and should be considered if staging investigations show evidence of dissemination. Local disease may respond if the tumour remains chemosensitive.

METASTATIC DISEASE

The pattern of survival in patients with metastatic disease is variable. Some patients with hormone sensitive disease have good long-term survival after sequential hormone manipulation. Patients with disease which is not hormone sensitive have much lower survival rates. The clinical pattern of relapse predicts future behaviour. Patients with a long disease-free interval (>2 years following primary diagnosis) and favourable sites of recurrence (such as bone, lymph nodes and chest wall) survive much longer than patients who have either a short disease-free interval or recurrence at other sites. Patients with lung, liver or brain disease have the poorest outlook.

Metastatic disease may be present at the time of diagnosis or may develop following primary treatment for operable breast cancer, either alone or in association with local recurrence.

The aim of treatment is to produce effective control of symptoms and prolong survival. The primary aim, however, is to improve quality of life. At the present time, there is no evidence that treating asymptomatic metastases improves survival and it is not appropriate to perform regular routine screening investigations for systemic disease during follow up. The choice of whether patients should have hormonal treatments or chemotherapy depends on the biology of the disease. Good prognosis disease is best treated by hormonal treatment, whereas poor prognosis disease usually requires chemotherapy (Fig. 7.2).

Hormonal treatment

A variety of hormonal agents are available for use in metastatic breast cancer. Although generally regarded as causing few side-effects, all therapies can cause distressing symptoms. Objective responses to hormonal agents are seen in 30% of all patients and in

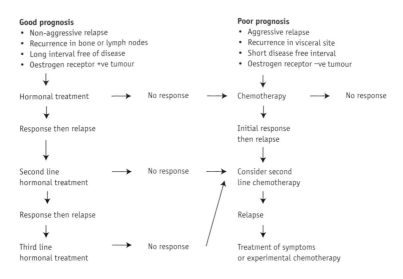

Fig. 7.2   Summary of treatment of metastatic disease.

50–60% of patients with ER-positive tumours. Response rates of 25% are seen with second line hormonal treatments, although less than 15% of patients who show no response to first line hormonal treatment, will respond to second line treatment, and 10–15% respond to third line treatment. Appropriate hormonal treatments for metastatic breast cancer are shown in Table 7.4.

Table 7.4   Hormonal treatment of metastatic breast cancer

Premenopausal patients
- 1st first line treatment:
  LHRH agonists if not previously used
  If patients had previous oophorectomy, LHRH agonists + tamoxifen

Postmenopausal patients
- 1st line treatment:
  Tamoxifen if not previously used or
  an aromatase inhibitor such as anastrozole or letrozole*

- 2nd line treatment:
  Following tamoxifen, anastrozole or letrozole*
  Following anastrazole or letrozole*, megestrol acetate

- Third line treatment
  Following anastrozole or letrozole*, progestogens

---

* further oral aromatase inhibitors will be available in the next two years

Chemotherapy

With chemotherapy, a balance has to be struck between achieving a high rate of response and limiting side-effects. The best palliation and subsequent quality of life is obtained with regimens which produce the highest response rates. Studies which have compared different intensities of chemotherapy show that quality of life is better on more intensive regimes with their associated side-effects, rather than with less intensive regimes which have lower response rates and fewer side-effects. Overall rates of response to chemotherapy are about 40–60% with a median time to relapse of 6–10 months. Subsequent courses of chemotherapy have low rates of response of less than 25%. The agents used for treating metastatic disease are similar to those in the adjuvant or primary systemic therapy settings.

Short-term results from high-dose chemotherapy with bone marrow or stem cell rescue for metastatic breast cancer appear promising. After 3–10 years, 15–20% of patients are disease free. One randomized study has shown a significant survival benefit for patients having stem cell rescue, but this study has been criticized, because the survival of patients given standard doses of chemotherapy was less than would have been expected. In addition, long-term tamoxifen was given only to the chemotherapy responders in a population of women that included a substantial number of ER-positive cancers. Larger long-term controlled studies of single and double dose intensity regimens with single or double stem cell rescues are currently underway.

ASSESSMENT OF RESPONSE

The commonly used outcome measures include relapse-free and overall survival. These are usually well defined but should be used in conjunction with some assessment of quality of life. The performance status (a crude measure of how well the patient is) is usually quoted on the Karnofsky or World Health Organization (WHO) score and can be used to see if treatment improves physical symptoms (Table 7.5).

Toxicity of treatments are well quantified using the WHO grades (Table 7.6) and should be used to specify toxicity in trials or new treatments. The median duration of response of any treatment is when 50% of patients treated have relapsed and gives some idea of efficacy.

The response of a tumour is generally given in terms of a complete response (CR), partial response (PR), disease stabilization (DS) and disease progression (DP). There are well-defined criteria for each grouping based on International Union against Cancer (UICC) guidelines. These can be found in any oncology text. They

Table 7.5 Performance status. Karnofsky and WHO grading

WHO criteria		Karnofsky	
0	Able to carry on normal activity	100	Normal; no complaints; no evidence of disease
		90	Able to carry on normal activity; minor signs of disease
1	Patient able to live at home tolerable tumour manifestation	80	Normal activity with effort; some signs and symptoms of disease
		70	Cares for self; unable to carry on normal activity
2	Patient with disabling tumour manifestations but <50% of time in bed	60	Requires occasional assistance but can care for most of her needs
		50	Requires considerable assistance and much medical care
3	Patient severely disabled and >50% of time in bed but able to stand up	40	Disabled; requires special care
		30	Severely disabled; hospitilization but death not imminent
4	Patient very sick and	20	Very sick; active support and bedridden; hospital treatment needed
		10	Moribund, fatal processes — progressing rapidly
5	Dead	5	Dead

are easier to apply when there is measurable disease such as a solitary metastasis but can be difficult to use if the disease is diffuse or if some areas are responding whilst others progress. With increasing use of primary systemic chemotherapy there is a need to assess the

Table 7.6 Simplified WHO grading system for toxicity of therapy

Grade	0	1	2	3	4
Haemoglobin	>11.0	9.5–11	8.0–9.4	6.5–7.9	<6.5g/dl
Leucocytes	>4.0	3.0–3.9	2.0–2.9	1.0–1.9	<1x10⁹/L
Platelets	>100	75–99	50–74	25–49	<25x10⁹/L
Nausea/ vomiting	None	Nausea	Transient vomiting	Therapy needed	Intractable
Hair loss	No change	Minimal	Patchy alopecia	Complete alopecia	Irreversible

change in size of a tumour in the treated breast. This can be done with ultrasound and an estimate of tumour volume can be obtained from three-dimensional measurements.

Patients who respond to therapy do better and can achieve long-term control of their disease. Those who do not respond need alternative therapies but rarely do so well.

SPECIFIC PROBLEMS SEEN IN PATIENTS WITH ADVANCED DISEASE

These include: hypercalcaemia; pathological fractures; pain; breathlessness from pleural or pulmonary disease, and raised intracranial pressure from cerebral secondaries.

Bone disease

Bone is the most common site of secondary breast cancer with three-quarters of patients having bone metastases. Widespread bone disease alone often responds well to hormonal treatment but when associated with visceral disease or if it occurs in young patients, chemotherapy is usually required. Assessing response to treatment is difficult and studies suggest that tumour markers may be of more use than repeated X-rays or bone scans. Most clinicians use control of symptoms to determine response to therapy.

Localized bone pain can be treated by a single fraction of radiotherapy. Widespread bone pain can be treated with radioactive strontium with few side-effects or with sequential upper and lower hemibody radiotherapy being an alternative. This latter treatment is associated with more toxicity. Bisphosphonates are useful for diffuse bone pain. Bisphosphonates may also be useful in preventing fractures and morbidity. Their role has been evaluated in one study which suggested that they were beneficial, but this needs to be confirmed in other studies. When bone lysis threatens fracture, internal fixation followed by radiotherapy (low doses in a few fractions) will improve quality of life and maintain mobility. Such treatment is often associated with a reasonable survival. If a pathological fracture does occur a combination of internal fixation and radiotherapy should be used although the functional result is usually inferior to that of prophylactic treatment. Detection of bone metastases can be a problem. Some patients have infiltration of marrow causing pain rather than bone destruction. Such disease is often best detected by MRI or computerized tomography (CT) scanning rather than by bone scanning or plain X-rays. Widespread marrow infiltration can cause a leuco-erythroblastic blood picture (immature cells in the peripheral blood). In such patients chemotherapy is generally required although it initially has to be given in reduced doses with careful monitoring and adequate supportive care.

Hypercalcaemia

These patients should be treated by hydration with saline (about 3 litres are given over 24 h) and intravenous bisphosphonates. Effective anticancer treatment reduces the risk of recurrence but patients who exhibit continuing hypercalcaemia can be treated with repeated intravenous bisphosphonates. Bisphosphonates restore normocalcaemia in 2–3 days but treatment may have to be repeated after a period varying between 2–3 weeks and 3 months to maintain this response unless the tumour responds to appropriate systemic therapy. They are usually given in the acute phase although maintenance therapy can be achieved by the oral route. Gut absorption does however remain a problem for bisphosphonates.

Malignant pleural effusion

Up to half of patients with metastatic breast cancer will develop a malignant pleural effusion and some of these require specific treatment. When examining the fluid aspirated, only 85% of patients actually have malignant cells in the effusion fluid. Although aspiration is effective at establishing a diagnosis, it is not an effective treatment. Tube drainage controls effusions in just over one-third of patients. For the other two-thirds who get recurrent effusions, installation of bleomycin, tetracycline or occasionally talc, inserted under general anaesthesia, is required to control recurrence. The effusion should be aspirated to complete dryness and then a small amount of local anaesthetic placed before adding the active agent. This reduces the pain associated with the procedure. Patients often develop transient pyrexial following this procedure.

The highest control rates are achieved by a combination of thoracoscopy, drainage of all the fluid under direct vision and insertion of talc. This requires a general anaesthetic but reduces the need for multiple aspirations and adds to the long-term quality of life.

Neurological complications

Although non-metastatic syndromes of the central nervous system (CNS) can occur with breast cancer, any focal neurological symptom must be investigated. CT or MRI can detect even small volumes of disease in the brain or spinal cord. Initial treatment of brain meta-stases is to reduce oedema with high-dose corticosteroids (dexam-ethasone 12–16 mg daily) pending local treatment with fractionated radiotherapy. Radiotherapy produces most benefit in patients whose neurological symptoms improve after taking steroids. Radiotherapy is delivered in five daily fractions. The long-term results of treating CNS disease are disappointing with most patients dying within 3–4 months. Long-term survival has been reported in patients with isolated brain metastases following excision of meta-stases and post-operative radiotherapy.

Cord compression is not usually amenable to surgery and is seen most often in patients with thoracic spinal metastases. Treatment is with steroids and fractionated radiotherapy. The treatment needs to be started as soon as possible and before any neurological deficits are severe. Occasionally patients do have isolated metastases caus-ing cord compression and in these patients laminectomy can be effective.

Cerebral metastases

These may cause distressing symptoms and are treated with dexam-ethasone (4 mg q.d.s.) to reduce the swelling that is often respons-ible for the symptoms. Occasionally craniotomy to excise a solitary metastasis is indicated but recurrence is common. Cranial radio-therapy can delay recurrence of symptoms if a good response to dex-amethasone is seen but is accompanied by side-effects of nausea and total alopecia. Even temporary restoration of normal faculties with these treatments is worthwhile, especially if this is the first sign of metastatic disease, as it may allow enough time for a patient to put their affairs in order.

SYMPTOM CONTROL AND PALLIATIVE CARE

Pain

Of patients with advanced breast cancer, 60–70% complain of pain. Patients with metastatic cancer rarely have only one pain and the majority have several separate pains which may have different causes. Each site of pain should be identified and the underlying mechanism determined if possible. It is important to appreciate that the patient's emotional state (anger, despair, fear, anxiety, depression) may be important in how the patient responds to their pain. It is useful, therefore, to assess both the physical and emotional aspects of the patient's pain. Three stages of pain control have been described:

- To be pain free at night.
- To be pain free at rest.
- To be pain free on movement.

While it is often possible to achieve the first two, the third may be difficult where there is widespread skeletal involvement. Analgesic approach to pain relief should be simple and flexible. Pain can be considered as mild, moderate and severe; appropriate treatments for these are outlined in Table 7.7.

Simple analgesics and opioids

Many patients do not receive an adequate trial of simple analgesics but, where they are ineffective, regular weak opioids such as co-proxamol or dihydrocodeine should be the next therapeutic step before proceeding to a strong opioid.

Strong opioid analgesics

Morphine remains the strong opioid analgesic of choice for severe pain. Dose requirements vary widely from one patient to another but the dose should be started low and titrated against the pain until control is achieved. During dose titration aqueous morphine elixir should be used because it has a rapid onset and a short duration of action, but once stable dose requirements have been determined controlled release preparations, such as morphine (slow release), given twice or three times daily, are more convenient and improve patient compliance. An identical daily dose of slow-release morphine (such as MST) should be substituted once the correct dose has been found. If breakthrough pain occurs during treatment with slow release preparations, morphine elixir can be added; although, if breakthrough pain is a frequent problem then the dose of MST should be increased.

Table 7.7 Choice of analgesic for pain control

Pain severity	Class of analgesic	Preferred drug
Mild pain	Simple analgesic	Paracetemol (preferable to aspirin because of lack of gastrointestinal side-effects)
Moderate pain	Weak opioid analgesic (alone or in combination with simple analgesic)	Co-proxamol or codeine + paracetemol
Severe pain	Strong opioid analgesic	Morphine

It should be appreciated that slow-release preparations should not be used for acute pain, as peak plasma concentrations of morphine are not reached for 2–4 h following administration. If medication cannot be given by mouth, rectal administration is an alternative route using the same dose and frequency as oral administration.

Parenteral opioids are not more effective than oral opioids although a smaller dose is required. The dose of oral morphine should be halved to give an equivalent dose of parenteral morphine. As diamorphine is more soluble than morphine, the dose of oral morphine should be divided by three to obtain an equivalent dose for parenteral administration. Morphine can be delivered subcutaneously using a continuous infusion pump.

None of the other strong opioid analgesics have advantages which make them preferable to morphine.

Side-effects of morphine

The common side-effects are drowsiness, constipation, nausea, vomiting and dry mouth. Drowsiness is usually only a problem at the start of treatment or when doses are increased; it usually resolves within a few days, when the dose has been stabilized. Constipation is a universal side-effect and all patients taking morphine should receive a regular laxative. Nausea and vomiting occur in one-half to two-thirds of patients, and the preferable antiemetic is haloperidol given once or twice daily in a dose of 1.5 mg. Respiratory depression and addiction do not occur in cancer patients.

Adjuvant drugs

These may not have intrinsic analgesic activity but contribute significantly to pain relief when used in combination with a conventional analgesic (Table 7.8). Anxiety, depression, fear, restlessness and insomnia can all significantly reduce a patient's pain threshold and these symptoms often respond to benzodiazepine medication. Diazepam is the preferred oral anxiolytic, temazepam the hypnotic of choice and midazolam the choice for parenteral use. This latter drug which can be given by subcutaneous infusion is particularly useful in the management of terminal restlessness. The place of antidepressants in the management of chronic pain is not clear but some patients with advanced or terminal malignant disease do appear to respond to them.

Table 7.8 Adjuvant drugs in pain control

Cause of pain	Useful adjuvant drugs
Bone pain	NSAIDs, bisphosphonates
Soft tissue infiltration	NSAIDs or steroids
Hepatic enlargement	Steroids
Raised intracranial pressure	Steroids
Nerve compression or infiltration	Steroids
	Amitriptyline
	Carbamazepine
	Mexiletine
Muscle spasm	Diazepam
	Baclofen
Fungating tumour	Antibiotics (metronidazole)
Cellulitis	Antibiotics

NSAIDs = non-steroidal anti-inflammatory drugs

Anticonvulsants are of value for lancinating or stabbing dysaesthetic pains associated with nerve infiltration or compression, postsurgical neuralgia, postherpetic neuralgia and other forms of neuropathic pain. Side-effects may be a problem with these drugs and so the initial dose should be low and titrated against the effects. The drug of choice is carbamazepine, initially starting at a dose of 100 mg twice a day and increasing to 800 mg per day.

Control of other symptoms (Table 7.9)

Table 7.9 Control of other symptoms in patients with metastatic breast cancer

Symptom	Treatment
Anorexia	Prednisolone or progestogens
Dysphagia	Antifungal drugs if related to candidiasis
	External beam irradiation, surgical intubation, or endoscopic laser treatment if mechanical evidence of obstruction
	Consider chemotherapy if dysphagia due to mediastinal node compression
Nausea and vomiting	Treat underlying cause
	Antiemetics (such as metoclopramide or cyclizine) with or without prednisolone
Constipation	Laxatives
Dyspnoea	Morphine and benzodiazepines
Cough	Codeine or methadone linctus or morphine oral solution
	Nebulized local anaesthetics

Lymphoedema

Upper limb lymphoedema is frequently encountered in patients with local recurrence in the axilla and supraclavicular regions. It may also occur as a complication of surgery or radiotherapy in the absence of local recurrence. It is a difficult problem to treat and often causes considerable pain and discomfort. In the first instance an elastic stocking or sleeve should be used in conjunction with other measures which include massage, limb exercise, compression bandaging and the use of intermittent compression sleeve devices.

Anorexia

Alcohol, corticosteroids and progestogens are the most helpful pharmacological treatments.

Dysphagia

This may occur because of oropharyngeal candidiasis or as a result of local tumour infiltration. The specific cause should therefore be sought. Treatment for candida includes nystatin suspension, amphotericin lozenges or fluconazole. External beam irradiation, surgical intubation or endoscopic laser therapy may be indicated where there is mechanical evidence of obstruction by tumour.

Nausea and vomiting

Nausea and vomiting may have many causes: drugs, uraemia, hepatic failure, hypercalcaemia, raised intracranial pressure and obstruction. Attention to the underlying cause and appropriate management with antiemetics is the mainstay of treatment.

Respiratory symptoms, lymphangitis carcinomatosa

Steroids are usually tried but are rarely effective. Non-specific symptomatic measures are the only option for the majority of patients.

Symptomatic treatment of dyspnoea

Morphine or other strong opioid drugs can give subjective relief for dyspnoea. Bronchodilators are only useful where reversible airways obstruction can be demonstrated. There is some anecdotal evidence to suggest that nebulized local anaesthetics may be useful in some patients. While having no specific effects on dyspnoea, reduction of the associated anxiety can be achieved using a small dose of benzo-diazopines. Oxygen is often used but has only a placebo effect.

Cough

This can be a difficult symptom to control. Opioid drugs remain the mainstay in the form of codeine linctus or morphine elixir. Troublesome cough can be helped by nebulized local anaesthetics such as marcaine.

Headache

In patients with advanced breast cancer, headache may have many causes, and migraine and tension headaches are probably more common than raised intracranial pressure associated with cerebral metastases.

If there are cerebral metastases they should be treated with a combination of cranial irradiation and dexamethasone 4 mg q.d.s.

Incontinence

There are a number of aids available to help with incontinence which reduces the distress that this causes.

Bone pain

Single fractions of radiotherapy to localized painful bony metastases are frequently effective. For more generalized bone pain, bisphos-phonates can, on occasion, produce symptomatic relief.

Malodour

Odour from fungating tumours, septic bedsores and incontinence due to poor laundry are an embarrassment for patients. Odour from fungating tumours and infected bedsores can often be controlled by the application of antibiotics such as metronidazole gel.

General considerations

Hospice care

Doctors and nurses involved in palliative care are experts in allevi-ating symptoms of terminal illness. Providing the patient and gen-eral practitioner are agreeable, the hospice team should be contacted as early as possible, once it is appreciated that the patient is enter-ing the terminal phase of their illness. It should be remembered that hospices can offer both outpatient as well as inpatient support, as well as having social workers with specific training in this area.

Terminal care

For the majority of patients who die from metastatic breast cancer, death is not a sudden event. During this period the aim of management is to maintain the patient in a comfortable and peaceful condition. Although oral medication is possible in the initial phase, there comes a time when, because of impaired consciousness, oral medication is no longer possible and should be changed to either the rectal or parenteral route.

Maintaining patients at home

Early domestic support from district nursing services or local hospice nurses is invaluable. Patients and their relatives should be made fully aware of the resources which are available in and out of the Health Service. These include Attendance Allowance (which can be made available speedily through the Special Rules) and various other allowances. Not enough consideration is given to financial implications; dying patients and their relatives should be put in touch with social workers and, where appropriate, local charities. Links to the hospital and primary care teams should be maintained to allow easy access if specific symptoms need addressing. The role of the MacMillan nurses in co-ordinating this phase is important.

It should also be appreciated that the carers themselves suffer physical symptoms looking after patients in the terminal phase of their disease and may also require support.

8. Breast reconstruction

Breast reconstruction used to be restricted to patients having a mastectomy — either as an immediate or as a delayed procedure. However, the use of a latissimus dorsi mini-flap allows a very wide excision with subsequent filling of the defect. The first question to ask, therefore, is whether a patient should proceed to mastectomy with immediate reconstruction or whether a very wide excision and partial reconstruction is possible. The latissimus flap procedure is also useful for the 15% of patients who have a poor cosmetic outcome following wide excision and radiotherapy. If a mastectomy has been performed then the purpose of breast reconstruction is to provide a breast mound with breast symmetry. In centres that provide reconstruction there has been a consistent increase in demand and up to one-half of patients offered immediate reconstruction take up this offer. Reconstruction may be immediate or delayed. Immediate reconstruction is less time consuming for the patient (but not for the surgeon) but care has to be taken that an oncological operation is not jeopardized for a better cosmetic result. Some would say that one surgeon should not perform both operations although these comments are heard most often in the USA where two surgeons means more money!

The choice of operation for an individual patient depends on several factors. Reconstruction can be carried out either by immediate placement of a prosthesis, usually in the subpectoral position, by placement of a tissue expander with subsequent stretching of the skin and muscle with eventual replacement of the expander with a prosthesis (silicone, saline or soya bean oil) or by a myocutaneous flap with or without a prosthesis. The two most common myocutaneous flaps require movement of either part of the latissimus dorsi muscle (Fig. 8.1) with overlying skin or the lower abdominal fat and skin based on the rectus abdominis muscle (Transverse Rectus Abdominis Myocutaneous flap [TRAM]) (Fig. 8.2). The latter may be carried out either as a rotational flap based on the superior epigastric artery or as

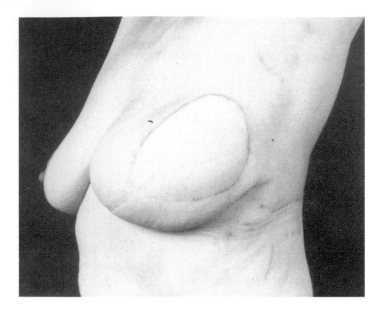

Fig. 8.1   Example of a latissimus dorsi rotational flap used for breast reconstruction.

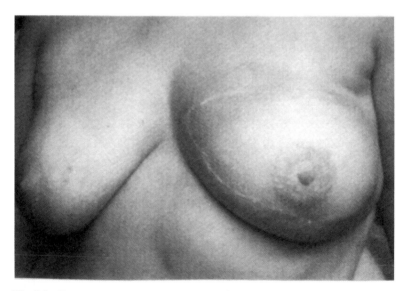

Fig. 8.2   Example of a TRAM flap reconstruction. Note subsequent nipple reconstruction.

a free flap using a microvascular anastamosis of the inferior epigastric vessels to the subscapular or thoracodorsal vessels. Choice depends on breast size, previous treatment and surgical expertise.

Options for breast reconstruction are outline in Table 8.1.

TISSUE EXPANSION AND SUBSEQUENT PLACEMENT OF PROSTHESIS

The scare about safety of silicone implants has put some women off having this technique. There are now other prostheses available including saline and soya bean oil. Saline implants were prone initially to leakage and deflation but the leak rate of prostheses available at the present time is much less. Breast prostheses are generally implanted after a period of tissue expansion (Fig 8.3). This involved placement of a plastic bag connected to a valve in a pocket created under the chest wall muscles (pectoralis major, parts of the serratus anterior, rectus abdominus and the external oblique).

Textured expanders (i.e. those with a ridged rather than smooth shell) are now available and seem to produce more rapid tissue expansion than smooth-walled expanders.

It is difficult to create large mounds by tissue expansion. If this technique is to be used in a patient with large breasts, the possibility of reducing the contralateral breast should be considered and discussed with the patient. A prosthesis that combines an expander with a definitive prosthesis is available and can be used for delayed reconstruction. It contains two cavities, one containing silicone gel and the other which can be inflated with saline. After over-inflation the volume of saline is reduced to obtain the desired volume; the port is then removed and the expander/prosthesis is left *in situ*.

Table 8.1 Options for breast reconstruction

Technique	Indications for immediate reconstruction	Indications for delayed reconstruction
Prosthesis	Small breasts Adequate skin flaps	As for immediate reconstruction plus Well healed scar plus no radiotherapy
Tissue expansion and prosthesis	Adequate skin flaps Good skin closure Small to medium breasts	As for immediate reconstruction plus no radiotherapy
Myocutaneous flaps	Large skin incision Doubtful skin closure Large breasts	As for immediate reconstruction Can be used if previous radiotherapy

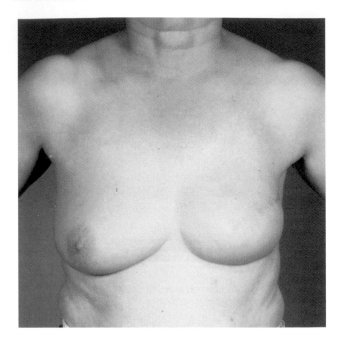

Fig. 8.3 Results of tissue expansion and then insertion of a prosthesis for breast reconstruction.

Myocutaneous flaps

Latissimus flaps usually require a prosthesis to be placed between them and the chest wall to create a breast mound. TRAM flaps are more bulky and have the advantage that they do not usually require the insertion of an implant.

Complications of breast surgery

Fibrous capsules occur around breast prostheses. Subsequent contraction of these capsules around the implant causes pain and an unsatisfactory shape. The use of textured prostheses has reduced the incidence of capsule contraction from over 50% with smooth implants at 1 year to less than 10%. Capsular contraction results in hardening and distortion of the reconstructed breast mound and often causes pain, discomfort and embarrassment. The treatment is capsulotomy either as a closed procedure or by capsular excision and replacement of a prosthesis with a textured implant (if a smooth implant has been used previously).

Infection

This occurs in about 5% of patients and means that the prosthesis has to be removed. Most units use prophylactic antibiotics to limit the rate of infection. Low-grade infection can occasionally manifest as early capsular contraction or erosion of the prosthesis through the overlying skin. The patient needs to be made aware of this 'complication' as well as the occasional haematoma which may require a return to theatre to drain.

Implant fatigue and rupture

This is a major concern among patients as it leads to leakage of silicone gel. The incidence of capsular rupture increases with time and is particularly common among early varieties with a thin shell. Ruptures are usually intracapsular and so the silicone does not usually leak into the body. All implants bleed a small amount of silicone but there is no evidence that leakage of silicone causes problems. In particular, women with implants do not seem to have a higher rate of connective tissue disorders (scleroderma, systemic lupus erythematosus, rheumatoid arthritis, etc.) than age-matched controls without implants. Few good studies of this subject have been performed and research is continuing. The lack of an association between silicone and connective tissue disorders is confirmed by the observation that other patients exposed to silicone (for example patients with silastic joints, heart valves containing silicone or siliconized arteriovenous shunts) do not have an excess of these disorders.

SUBCUTANEOUS MASTECTOMY

Patients with extensive DCIS or those having a prophylactic mastectomy may be offered a subcutaneous mastectomy with immediate placement of a subcutaneous prosthesis. This used to be unsatisfactory due to capsular contracture, which was easily seen when the prosthesis was just below the skin. This has been remedied to some extent by the use of textured surface prostheses (Fig. 8.4). Some surgeons have used a period of tissue expansion to try and achieve a better final cosmetic outcome. A newer technique reconstructing the breast with a de-epithelialized TRAM flap gives the most natural and aesthetically pleasing result. Subcutaneous mastectomy removes the majority of breast tissue but care has to be taken in planning incisions as there may be a problem in reaching all the breast tissue and, if the patient has already had a biopsy, areas of poor vascularity may result. A pad under the nipple is often left to preserve its blood supply but, even so, nipple necrosis is a potential complication. A biopsy of the pad under the nipple must be taken to ensure malignant cells are not present. Patients need to be aware that cancer can develop or recur under the nipple and that it may need resection at a later date.

NIPPLE RECONSTRUCTION

The final touch after breast reconstruction. This can be carried out by a number of surgical techniques. Some require transplantation of darker skin (common donor sites being the skin behind the ear or from the labia) whereas others create a nipple using the skin of the breast and tattoo the skin to achieve a colour match. That there are so many techniques available is a reflection of how unsatisfactory many are in the long term.

Another technique is to use a stick-on nipple which can be removed and worn by the patient at her will. The commercial varieties are unrealistic but it is possible to make a customized nipple by taking a plaster cast impression of the remaining side. A colour-matched silastic prosthesis is then made and is more realistic (Fig. 8.5) and carries greater patient acceptability (Fig. 8.6).

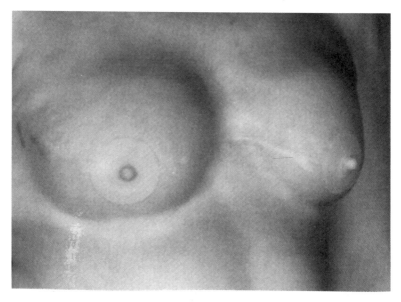

Fig. 8.6   A patient wearing her false reconstruction. (Reproduced with permission from Sainsbury et al 1991 Ann Roy Coll Surg Engl 73: 67–69.)

9. Clinical trials

The use of clinical trials has provided the information upon which a logical treatment for breast cancer can be based and future trials planned. An overview of randomized clinical trials in breast cancer was held in Oxford in 1990 and again in 1995. The 1990 results were published in the Lancet in early 1992 and confirmed that adjuvant chemotherapy provides major benefits for premenopausal woman as does adjuvant tamoxifen for the postmenopausal woman. This review of 75 000 women from 133 randomized trials contained data based on 31 000 recurrences and 24 000 deaths. The results from the 1995 overview are awaited in publication form although preliminary release of the data has shown a benefit for tamoxifen for premenopausal women as well, but with a lower success rate.

The history of trials can be divided into three eras. The early trials were basically of more versus less surgery and/or radiotherapy. An example of this was the Kings/Cambridge trial of adjuvant radiotherapy. Then came the trials of less surgery versus standard mastectomy such as the NSABP B-06 (National Surgical Adjuvant Breast and Bowel Project). Finally the era of large trials on the role of chemotherapy and endocrine therapy came in. The NATO (Nolvadex Adjuvant Trial Organisation) trial which randomized postmenopausal patients to 2 years tamoxifen versus no adjuvant treatment typifies this era.

The future of trials is improving as their importance is recognized and funding for their running is provided. At one stage less than 2% of eligible patients were entered into a clinical trial. Reasons given included clinicians' disinclination, pressure of work or because the patient refused randomization. There is evidence that patients in trials receive better treatment and may survive longer. With appropriate support (data management and research nurses) and a profile of trials to catch most patients some centres are now reporting greater than 80% trial entry.

The recent introduction of Regional Ethics Committees may reduce some of the frustrations of trying to run multicentre trials which were subject to the whims of local ethics committees even after national approval.

The UKCCCR (United Kingdom Co-ordinating Committee for Cancer Research) has a breast subgroup responsible for collating major trials in the UK. They do not provide financial support but act as a central co-ordinating group with representatives from the grant-giving bodies such as the Medical Research Council, Cancer Research Campaign and Imperial Cancer Relief Fund.

Some of the major trials currently underway (excluding industry-sponsored phase III studies) in the UK include:

Trials of primary medical therapy

TOPIC — infusional chemotherapy versus standard intravenous treatment.

Trials of high-dose chemotherapy for high-risk patients

Anglo-Celtic — for high-risk women. Conventional high-dose chemotherapy with or without a stem cell transplant.
ABO-1 — the use of taxoids in the adjuvant, high risk setting.

Trials of chemo-/endocrine therapy

ABC — a catch-all trial randomizing patients to chemotherapy or ovarian ablation (if premenopausal), all patients receiving tamoxifen.
NEAT — examination of the role of anthracyclines in the adjuvant setting.

Trials of endocrine therapy duration

ATTOM and ATLAS — both trials of tamoxifen duration.

Trials of adjuvant endocrine therapy

ATAC — aromatase inhibition with anastrazole versus tamoxifen alone or in combination.

Trials of special types of breast cancer

DCIS — role of radiotherapy and/or tamoxifen in completely excised DCIS.

BASO II — role of radiotherapy and/or tamoxifen in the management of small, special types of breast cancer.

Trials of prevention

IBIS — 5 years tamoxifen or placebo for prevention.

Studies of timing of surgery

ITS — Intervention, Timing and Survival study — looking at timing of surgery within menstrual cycle.

Psychology and breast disease

10. Psychological factors in patients with breast disease

INTRODUCTION

Breasts are not primarily sexual organs but are designed for feeding the young. This physiological fact is eclipsed by the emotional and cultural values placed on the breast which minimizes its basic function and emphasizes femininity and sexuality. The male subjected to the same influences also has a culturally determined interest in female breasts.

In light of the above, it is not surprising that many women have concerns about the size, shape and appearance of their breasts ranging from minor dissatisfaction to major preoccupation and anxiety. These concerns explain why the breast is second only to the nose as a focus for cosmetic surgery. Cultural considerations therefore have to be taken into account when assessing and treating breast disease.

BREAST CANCER

Discovering a breast lump is, understandably, an alarming experience, and even when this is found to be benign many women remain distressed. Some will go on to develop clinically significant mood illnesses, particularly if chronic mastalgia is a feature. So it is important not to dichotomize along the line that breast cancer means psychological problems and that no cancer means no problem. Nevertheless cancers of the breast clearly have the most important psychological concomitants.

It is convenient to consider these aspects under four main areas: antecedents; reactions to disease and treatment; factors in determining outcome, and counselling techniques and problems.

ANTECEDENTS

This issue is bedevilled by the variable and indeterminable lag between tumour onset and the presentation of the patient. Also, breast tumours may grow at varying and uneven rates and patients present at different stages, so distinguishing antecedents from reactions can prove difficult. Most studies have employed a cross-sectional design, often a single assessment at or shortly after presentation when the patient knows or suspects their diagnosis — which may bias their recollections and responses. Antecedents include mental illness, adverse life effects and cancer-prone personality (type C personality).

Mental illness

Depression as a potential precursor of cancer is an unresolved issue with evidence for a weak association in epidemiological research but conflicting findings in smaller studies of affected patients. The likelihood of a patient with breast cancer having had a depressive illness treated during the preceding 5 years is no greater than for matched controls with benign breast disease.

Life events and stresses

Again, epidemiological studies tend to show a weak association between stressful events and the onset of cancer; but there is no evidence of an association between the diagnosis of breast cancer and preceding stressful life events of any severity, recent or remote, when affected women are compared with matched women who have benign breast disease.

Cancer-prone personality

It is possible that certain personality attributes may predispose women to breast cancer. The studies all have weaknesses and a valid relationship has not been firmly established, but there are impressively consistent differences reported in personality traits between women with breast cancer and those with benign or no breast disease. These findings refer particularly to patients under 50 years of age and have also been reported less frequently in other female cancers.

The main personality traits, termed variously type C or cancer-proneness, cluster round an inability to master anger which is expressed, for instance, as an excessive suppression of anger and an enhanced tendency to avoid conflicts. Low anxiousness is also described. Such women respond to stress by using a repressive coping style, i.e. they don't let their feelings show, a core facet which has been termed 'repressive defensiveness'. How this might be transduced into cancer-proneness is uncertain.

Managing the issue of control over cancer

The prospect that, for some patients, there are factors within their own character that may have contributed to the development of their breast tumour, can prove frightening or invigorating; and the doctor faced with a patient who is knowledgeable or curious about this must recognize this is a double-edged weapon that needs to be handled carefully.

Part of the polarization of views that sometimes arises between the patient and doctor occurs because doctors may either not fully appreciate the psychological attitudes of their patient or regard such ideas as competitive with their own: so instead of psychological interventions being regarded as complimentary, they become alternative. There would be less rejection of orthodox medicine if these aspects and needs of the patient were taken into account.

REACTIONS

These include reactions to breast cancer, surgery and adjuvant treatments.

Breast cancer

Prevalence and morbidity

The prevalence of psychological disorders in the year following diagnosis of breast cancer has consistently been reported around 30%, which is three to four times what would be expected in the general population. Most patients carry a diagnosis of anxiety and/or depressive illness. These are typically mild disorders and, indeed, severe illnesses are only slightly more frequent than expected.

With such high levels of morbidity it may seem surprising that referral rates for psychological help are low; for instance the first 50 referrals from a breast cancer unit specialist liaison service were gleaned from around 3000 patients, i.e. only about 1.7% of patients were referred.

There are a number of explanations for low levels of referral, but the discrepancy has been mainly attributed to medical factors in the consultation process:

- Failure to be empathic.
- Failure to ask questions about the patient's well-being, emotional state, attitudes and concerns in a manner that facilitates disclosure of problems.
- Failure to recognize the significance of these problems when they are disclosed, or to respond appropriately.

This is compounded by the reluctance of many patients to disclose how they feel unless they are positively encouraged to do so, for reasons such as not wanting to burden the doctor or fear of being considered inadequate.

On the other hand, it has been proposed that most of the 30% of cases reflect pseudomorbidity rather than true illness: indeed even with a mere 1.7% referral rate, the breast liaison service still reported that half of their patients had transient psychological reactions that required no more than brief counselling.

Adjustment reactions

For most women the threats, fears and losses associated with a breast lump, cancer and its treatment concern not just their health and survival, but their body image, sexuality and self-esteem, as well as their marriage, family life, work and social pursuits. These are not trivial matters and the emotional responses reflect the gravity of the situation.

Modulating thoughts, feelings and behaviours to cope with crisis is not a pathological process, rather it represents an adaptive response preparing the individual to adjust. Adjustment processes can become maladaptive either in degree, when an emotional illness requiring treatment develops, or in form, with abnormal coping responses such as extreme denial, deliberate self-harm, eating disorders, drug or alcohol abuse. However getting things out of proportion or going off the rails is usually something the patient, her family and/or her regular medical attendants recognize; and it is with the patient, supported and guided by others who know her, that the decision about the need for psychological intervention should rest, not with the presence of tears or a result on a psychiatric research scale.

Further, diagnosing mental disorder and prescribing treatment inappropriately is not harmless, especially if this is at variance with the patient's perspective. Adding the stigma of being a psychiatric patient to already distressing circumstances is one consequence; another is the generation of anxiety and misery through sentiments like 'something else is going wrong with me' and 'I ought to have been able to cope with this'.

The nurse counsellor

The majority of the 30% of patients who are classified as suffering from psychological morbidity do not need, and would not benefit from, psychiatric referral. They are suffering from appropriate emotional reactions which usually respond well to brief intervention, often only one or two counselling sessions being required. This is best portrayed as part of the disease process and handled by the surgical team, with the nurse counsellor/clinical nurse specialist/breast care nurse being pivotal in this regard. Recent research endorses her value, confirming that support from a breast care nurse was more effective at reducing psychological morbidity/distress among women with breast cancer than routine care from ward staff or support from a voluntary organization. Monitoring each patient once within 2 months of discharge is as effective as regular reviews, as patients will typically contact the nurse when they regard it as necessary, mainly to seek information or reassurance about their treatment.

This nurse requires psychological training, support and back-up, and ought to have good links with the liaison psychiatry service. The psychiatric service's role is to discuss those cases of concern to the nurse specialist, reviewing patients who are considered to be experiencing unusual, or unduly severe or prolonged symptoms, as well as those who have frank mental disorder.

Surgical treatment

For many patients it is the treatment rather than the disease which turns out to be the more unpleasant and distressing aspect. In the quest for prolonging survival or cure doctors have, in the past, underestimated the effects that their work has upon the patient. Now increasing attention is being paid to the quality of life associated with cancer treatments.

Some of the findings concerning psychological responses to different surgical techniques may prove surprising, and notably the discovery that emotional distress and psychological maladjustment is as frequent after lumpectomy as following mastectomy. The explanation appears to be that the removal of a breast leads to grieving for loss while conservation provokes mistrust about that breast with a fear that cancer is still lurking and a mastectomy will prove inevitable. However breast conservation (or immediate reconstruction) does reduce psychiatric morbidity among women who are particularly concerned about their appearance at the time of surgery. Also, mastectomized women tend to have lower self-esteem, greater social withdrawal and more frequent sexual dysfunction compared with women whose breast is retained.

Indeed sexual problems develop frequently after surgery, being disclosed by about one-third of patients, with the most common feature being loss of libido. Sexual dysfunction is reported nine times more frequently among women with body image dissatisfaction compared with women who find their appearance acceptable.

Given the choice, two-thirds of women in one study opted for mastectomy rather than lumpectomy, essentially to get the business over and done with. Just over one-half of patients in another study wanted the surgeon to decide their treatment without playing an active role. The likelihood of developing anxiety or depression was significantly greater among those patients treated by surgeons who favoured mastectomy and who did not offer a choice. The solution should be a 'horses for courses' approach, recognizing that some patients want to exercise choice while others do not, and that when survival is not materially affected, it is the patient's preference, if she has one, rather than surgical fashion that should be directive. If she has no preference then breast conservation is psychologically preferable because lumpectomy definitely wins over mastectomy in respect of satisfaction with body image.

Of course breast reconstruction with a prosthetic implant following mastectomy offers a means of resolving these conflicting emotional reactions in that the fear of cancer is removed without destroying physical integrity to the same extent. This procedure does improve satisfaction with body image compared with mastectomy, but with immediate reconstruction at least, beneficial effects upon emotional morbidity are not evident. It may be that better technology and timing of implant surgery will improve the psychological outcome, for these procedures still present problems in the frequency of surgical complications and subjective dissatisfaction with the cosmetic outcome.

Adjuvant treatment

- Chemotherapy causes considerable psychological morbidity, especially with prolonged courses of treatment. Because the cancer has been removed surgically and the patient perceives no immediate benefit from this additional therapy, its side-effects and disruption to life are even harder to tolerate than when chemotherapy is first line treatment. Conditioned vomiting or severe nausea develops in about one-quarter of patients to a degree that treatment is warranted.
- Radiotherapy can prove distressing for a few patients and is associated with increased physical symptoms and social dysfunction during the course, but not with greater anxiety or depression.

- Tamoxifen does not appear to be associated with adverse psychological effects.
- Depression may be more frequent after oophorectomy.

Finally, chemotherapy and radiotherapy are not associated with increased psychiatric morbidity once the course of treatment is completed.

VULNERABILITY FACTORS

Which women are most at risk of developing psychiatric morbidity? Vulnerability factors include general factors which predispose women to emotional illness and factors specific to breast cancer and its treatment.

General factors include:

- A previous history of psychiatric disorder (especially mood illness).
- An unsatisfactory or broken marriage.
- The lack of a confiding relationship.
- Major life stresses of an unwelcome nature.

Specific factors include:

- Lymphoedema or pain.
- Problems with body image.
- Oophorectomy.
- Chemotherapy, when the additional risk is confined to active therapy.

To this list should now be added health professional variables:

- The inability to communicate effectively.
- The failure to offer choice.

Family factors

Perhaps unexpectedly, being unmarried is protective among women with breast cancer, which probably reflects the special influence this form of cancer can have on a marriage. It is established that the husbands of breast cancer patients suffer physical symptoms and psychological distress, and for some loving and otherwise confiding partners the only way they can cope is by denial or some other maladaptive mechanism. Maladjustment in the spouse can add to the patient's guilt and fear, especially in a previously sound relationship. In these circumstances sexual dysfunction is particularly common and distressing — and compounds the problem. The impact of cancer upon the family unit is a complex, important issue, which has been sorely neglected compared with concern for the individual patient.

OUTCOME

The evidence that psychological factors contribute significantly to outcome, both in terms of mortality and relapse, is more compelling than for tumour genesis. Findings include mental illness, life events/stresses, personality and attitude/coping styles.

Mental illness

There is good evidence from a number of studies that women who are classified as psychiatric cases pre-operatively have a better chance of disease-free survival at 5 and more years. Bearing in mind the distinction made between a case on a research scale and clinical practice, it is probably safer to interpret this finding as meaning that it is women who are distressed at the time of diagnosis or surgery who have a better prognosis, rather than those who are suffering from a true mental illness.

Life events and stresses

There is mounting evidence, although still disputed, that severe adverse life events may predispose to or precipitate relapse.

Personality

There is evidence that women with breast cancer who have type C personality traits or cope through repressive defensiveness are more likely to relapse compared with women who are not. This ties in neatly with the mental illness findings, as type C individuals tend to report or convey less distress, anxiety and depression.

Attitudes/coping style

The best evidence that psychological features are independent mediators of disease-free survival comes from a study of only 57 patients first assessed in 1971 before biologically sophisticated measures such as hormone receptor status were widely available. The method involved the patient's coping style being delineated by the investigator on verbatim statements and current mood 3 months after simple mastectomy with attribution to one of four mutually exclusive categories:

- Denial (apparent active rejection of any evidence about the diagnosis which might have been offered).
- Fighting spirit (a highly optimistic attitude accompanied by a search for greater information about breast cancer).
- Stoic acceptance (acknowledgement of the diagnosis without enquiry for further information unless new symptoms developed).
- Feelings of helplessness/hopelessness (complete engulfment by knowledge of the diagnosis).

Five years later, patients who had been categorized as 'fighters' and 'deniers' were five to six times more likely to be surviving without recurrence compared with patients who had stoically accepted their lot or had decompensated into a helpless/hopeless state. This effect was maintained 10 and 15 years after assessment and could not be attributed to any crucial biological differences among the groups. Later studies from the UK, USA and Canada have confirmed that deniers and fighters have a greater chance of disease-free survival when compared with other attitudes. The scale of this effect appears to be large, but its explanation remains obscure. Potential explanations involve relationships between psychological state and concentrations of immunoglobulins, natural killer cells, prolactin and tumour oestrogen and progesterone status.

COUNSELLING AND PSYCHOSOCIAL INTERVENTIONS

There is a huge range of psychosocial interventions on offer to patients with cancer. A recent review of the literature focusing on the four mainstream interventions — behavioural therapy, educational therapy, psychotherapy and support groups — shows increasing evidence of efficacy. This was confirmed by a recent meta-analysis of 62 studies comparing treatment and control groups for various psychosocial, behavioural and psycho-educational approaches. Significant benefit was demonstrated in emotional adjustment, functional adjustment and symptoms related to the disease, but not for medical outcome.

The counselling process

Apart from the aims of information-giving, empathic support and the opportunity for ventilation, it is important to try to ascertain the personal meaning to a woman both of the disease itself and the treatment.

The disease

The term cancer has different meanings to different people depending on previous experience and fantasies. For example:

- Inevitable pain or death.
- Humiliation, shame, loss of dignity.
- Loss of control.

It is important to investigate ideas and beliefs about cancer and also to enquire about friends or relatives who have had cancer.

Women may feel that their bodies have betrayed them or are running amok, and may feel extremely concerned by any minor physical ailments, worrying that these may herald a recurrence. Women can also feel their bodies to be extremely vulnerable, as if the boundaries between inside and outside have been weakened. This may affect their ability to partake in physical exercise, or even to venture into places where there may be accidental physical contact such as busy shopping centres.

The treatment

The breast is intimately bound up with femininity, sexuality and creativity. It may be that loss of, or perceived disfigurement of, the breast may be more distressing to a woman than actually having cancer itself. This is particularly likely if a woman's self-esteem is tied up with her appearance and sexual identity.

Mastectomy, oophorectomy and the use of anti-oestrogen drugs can all be perceived as an attack on femininity, which may provoke resentment and non-compliance with treatment. Another possible outcome is that the patient may no longer feel that she has 'permission' to be a woman which can lead to sexual difficulties. Exploration of these issues may prove beneficial especially if the woman can be made aware of the reasons behind her reactions.

Chemotherapy and radiotherapy can cause a great deal of physical suffering and women often find themselves resenting the treatment but find it difficult to express angry feelings towards the doctors who are trying to help them. Patients also find it hard to tolerate the physical side-effects when there is no guarantee that the treatment will be effective.

Problems which can arise during counselling

Things can go wrong if a patient uses defence mechanisms excessively or if something happens to cause relationship difficulties between patient and counsellor. This usually happens because of transference or countertransference reactions. These terms will be explained below.

Common psychological reaction to loss

Of course not all women with breast cancer will experience severe difficulties but some psychological adjustment is invariably necessary.

Shock, anger, depression and acceptance all have their place when coming to terms with any loss and in fact are necessary. They will be recognizable to anyone working with bereaved patients or those who have been bereaved themselves. A patient does not work her way steadily through these feelings but will oscillate between them, gradually progressing towards acceptance.

Previous coping styles can provide some indication of how a woman is going to respond. Women who have been compulsively self-reliant may find it difficult to relinquish control to doctors and also find fighting an invisible enemy a problem. Previously dependent patients may be easier to deal with as they find the regression to patient status easier, although they may become excessively dependent on those treating them.

Commonly used psychological defence mechanisms

Defence mechanisms are universal and are unconscious 'mental tricks' which are used to avoid anxiety and mental pain. The following are both illustrative and commonly encountered among patients suffering from breast cancer and also dying patients:

- Denial — seeming not to be aware of diagnosis or prognosis; not a problem unless of such a degree that it prevents a patient from seeking proper treatment.
- Regression — reverting to a more child-like state; useful during acute illness but can be a problem during rehabilitation.
- Displacement — transferring feelings which belong to one person or situation on to another; e.g. anger with a doctor for late diagnosis may be inappropriately felt towards a spouse.
- Projection — feelings which really belong to oneself are projected on to others; e.g. a woman might unconsciously feel disgusted with her own body but projects that on to others so thinking that they find her disgusting.

Transference

This term means the development of feelings by the patient towards the therapist which really belong to important figures from the patient's past — usually parents. This usually aids treatment as it fosters trust and compliance. If however a patient has had a difficult relationship with her parents then this may be re-enacted with her therapist or doctor. She may complain that he/she is cold, uncaring or cruel. Recognizing that these feelings belong to the past and, if necessary, exploring them with the patient, can prevent serious breakdown in communications.

Countertransference

This refers to those feelings that a patient stirs up in her therapist and can be a form of unconscious communication. For example, a doctor may feel unaccountably despairing or overwhelmed when faced with a particular patient. If these are unusual feelings for him/her it is possible that the patient is communicating her own feelings about having cancer. Alternatively a therapist may feel unreasonably angry or irritable. Sensitive therapists can use these feelings to explore further how their patients really feel and, if they show that they can tolerate them, this does bring great feelings of relief.

Of course feelings can also originate in the therapist who has their own wealth of life experiences, defences and ways of dealing with situations. However, if the feelings engendered by a patient within the therapist are particularly uncomfortable, strong or uncharacteristic they should be considered as a potential communication of how that patient is feeling.

Psychotherapy with the dying patient

When a patient is dying the defence mechanisms of denial and regression are commonly brought into play and are extremely effective in aiding the patient to make the most of the end of her life and to die peacefully. Women who are experiencing excessive anxiety or depression often benefit from a bolstering of these defences, and this can be enhanced by the therapeutic use of transference. So if a patient feels that someone is concerned and caring for them in a maternal way they feel protected and are able to regress which can reinforce denial. Trust in the therapist is essential for this to occur, and trust is fostered by the therapist answering questions honestly, and being reliable and consistent in his/her approach to the patient. These therapist characteristics foster positive feelings in the patient which resemble previous infantile feelings towards her mother.

This is a time when patients need to feel that they are being listened to so it is better not to feel pressured to 'do' something. Most anxieties about dying are not existential in nature but are to do with the manner of dying. Reassurance about pain relief and alleviation of other physical symptoms is immensely comforting.

Monitoring the countertransference can be a useful guide to a patient's state of mind. Working with the dying can be enormously stressful because it stirs up feelings and fantasies that the therapist has about his/her own mortality and any previous personal experience of death. Defence mechanisms help deal with this, but sometimes if they become too effective, the therapist will be perceived as cold and remote; alternatively the therapist may become over-identified with the patient, recognizing aspects of him/herself in her, and then the therapist may be perceived as oppressive, intrusive and interfering.

Usually different patients stir up different feelings in a therapist, but if a therapist's response has become habitual it may be worth self-examination as this will probably be impeding therapeutic effectiveness.

BREAKING BAD NEWS

There is no easy way to break bad news however it is important to do it in such a way that the patient can bear the news, receive the information that she needs to know and to enable her to express her feelings and concerns.

The immediate impact

Upon learning that she has breast cancer a woman is liable to feel a number of complex emotions. These may be mitigated if the patient is asked to bring along a close relative or friend, as this has been shown to reduce depression, anxiety and improve adjustment 1 year later.

A friendly and unhurried interview with no interruptions will help. Be prepared for this meeting, martialling the facts, prioritizing the information that is to be given and considering appropriate responses to anticipated questions. Allow the patient time to react to the news without rushing in prematurely with reassurance or advice.

Be guided by the patient who will use verbal and non-verbal cues to indicate how much information she requires at the time.

Improving the information-giving process

Improved communication between doctors and their patients leads to better treatment compliance, improved trust and less likelihood

of litigation. An essential aspect of communication is that of information giving. Of 101 women with the diagnosis of early breast cancer
who were interviewed following the 'bad news' interview, over one-
half expressed dissatisfaction, feeling that the information they had
been given was inadequate. Surveys have shown that half the information given to patients is forgotten and 50% of patients would like
to ask questions but feel inhibited.

Ways to improve recall:

- Use the primary effect — patients remember information at the
  beginning of the interview better; therefore try to give the most
  important information first.
- Keep things simple — use short sentences, repetition and avoid
  medical terminology.
- Ask the patient to feedback what she has learned during the
  consultation.
- Use written information.
- Consider using other aids such as audiotapes of the consultation
  which the patient can then take home to replay.

Aiding the expression of emotions and concerns

As a profession, doctors tend to undervalue the benefits of listening
to patients and trying to understand their concerns. This is of great
benefit to the patient so it is worth trying not to succumb to the
temptation to falsely reassure or give advice straightaway, as these
measures more often reduce the doctor's own discomfort rather
than the patient's.

People in the caring professions desire to alleviate the suffering
of others. This can create problems when treating patients with cancer as doctors may feel anger, hopelessness or despair at their limited effectiveness. The reactions to these uncomfortable feelings may
include avoidance of emotional issues, false cheerfulness and optim-
ism, and concentration on purely physical aspects of the disease —
which may leave the patient feeling bewildered, isolated and
anxious.

To try to minimize these problems a practitioner needs to be
aware that he/she may feel uncomfortable with cancer patients for a
number of reasons, but problems can be avoided with some degree
of self-awareness. Practitioners working with cancer patients need
support for themselves (either formal or informal) and should seek
supervision from a mental health professional if they feel that they
are out of their depth. Once a patient feels confident that her doctor

can tolerate her difficult emotions and is not going to be over-whelmed, she will automatically feel more understood and will find this reassuring in itself.

Other approaches

A recent study shows that about 16% of patients use complementary therapies. The most popular are healing, relaxation, visualization, diets, homeopathy, vitamins, herbalism and the Bristol approach. Benefits of these therapies appear to be largely psychological. Patients using these therapies tend to be less satisfied with conventional treatment largely because of side-effects and lack of hope of cure. This study reinforces the belief that for many cancer patients hope is an important issue and hence it is important for doctors and nurses to establish good communication and maintain a hopeful attitude thereby fostering a more collaborative approach to management. The polarization of views that sometimes arises between the patient and her doctor occurs because the doctor either does not appreciate the psychological attitudes of their patient or regards such ideas as competitive with their own: so instead of non-conventional interventions being regarded as complementary they become alternative, when the patient's response is to eschew or become suspicious of orthodox medicine.

CONCLUSION

Taking account of the human experience is an essential ingredient of successfully managing disease. This chapter is not about how to become a popular doctor, it's about how to be a clinically more effective doctor through appreciating the psychological dimensions and the basics of skilful communication.

Further reading

The Breast Surgeons Group of the British Association of Surgical Oncology 1995 Guidelines for surgeons in the management of symptomatic breast disease in the United Kingdom. Eur J Surgical Oncol 21 (suppl A): 1–13

Bland KI, Copeland EM 1991 The breast. Comprehensive management of benign and malignant diseases. WB Saunders, Philadelphia

Bostwick J III 1990 Plastic and reconstructive breast surgery. Quality Medical Publications, St Louis, Missouri

Report of a working party of the British Breast Group 1994 Provision of breast services in the UK: The advantages of specialist units

Collaborative Group on Hormonal Factors in Breast Cancer 1997 Breast cancer and hormone replacement therapy: collaborative reanalysis of data from 51 epidemiological studies of 52, 705 women with breast cancer and 108, 411 women without breast cancer. Lancet 350: 1047–1059

de Moulin D 1989 A short history of breast cancer. Kluwer Academic Publishers, Dordrect, Germany

Dixon JM (ed.) 1995 ABC of breast disease. BMJ Publications, London

Early Breast Cancer Trialists' Collaborative Group 1992 Systemic treatment of early breast cancer by hormonal, cytotoxic or immune therapy. 133 randomised trials involving 31,000 recurrences and 24,000 deaths among 75,000 women. Lancet 339: 1–15, 71–85

Early Breast Cancer Trialists' Collaborative Group 1996 Ovarian ablation in early breast cancer: overview of the randomised trials. Lancet 348: 1189–96

Expert Advisory Group on Cancer to the Chief Medical Officers of England and Wales 1994 A policy framework for commissioning cancer services: a consultative document

Fallowfield U, Baum M 1984 Psychological welfare of patients with breast cancer. J R Soc Med 82: 4–5

Forrest P 1990 Breast cancer: the decision to screen. Nuffield Provincial Hospital Trust, London

Galea MH, Blamey RW, Elston CE, & Ellis IO 1992 The Nottingham prognostic index in primary breast cancer. Breast Cancer Res Treat 22: 207–219

Greer HS, Morris T, Pettingale KW 1979 Psychological response to breast cancer: effect on treatment. Lancet ii: 785–787

Harris JR, Lippman ME, Morrow M, & Hellman S 1996 Diseases of the breast. Lippincott-Raven, Philadelphia, New York

Hughes LE 1989 Progress symposium – Benign breast disorders: fibrocystic disease? or non disease? or ANDI. World J Surg 13: 667–764

Hughes LE, Mansel RE, Webster DJT 1989 Benign disorders and diseases of the breast. Balliere Tindall, London

Ley P 1988 Communicating with patients. Croom Helm, London

Page DL, Anderson TJ 1988 Diagnostic histopathology of the breast. Churchill Livingstone, Edinburgh

Powles TJ, Smith IE 1991 Medical management of breast cancer. Martin Dunitz, London

Ramirez A 1984 Liason psychiatry in a breast cancer unit. J R Soc Med 82: 15–17

Stewart HJ, Anderson TJ, Forrest APM 1991 Breast disease: new approaches. Br Med Bull 47: 251–522

Index